Birthrights

A Parents' Guide to Modern Childbirth

Sally Inch

HUTCHINSON

London Melbourne Sydney Auckland Johannesburg

Hutchinson & Co. (Publishers) Ltd
An imprint of the Hutchinson Publishing Group
17–21 Conway Street, London W1P 6JD

Hutchinson Group (Australia) Pty Ltd
30–32 Cremorne Street, Richmond South, Victoria 3121
PO Box 151, Broadway, New South Wales 2007

Hutchinson Group (NZ) Ltd
32–34 View Road, PO Box 40–086, Glenfield, Auckland 10

Hutchinson Group (SA) Pty Ltd
PO Box 337, Bergvlei 2012, South Africa

First published 1982
© Sally Inch 1982

Phototypeset in Linotron Plantin
by Input Typesetting Ltd, London

Printed in Great Britain by The Anchor Press
and bound by Wm Brendon & Son Ltd,
both of Tiptree, Essex

British Library Cataloguing in Publication Data

Inch, Sally
  Birthrights.
  1. Childbirth at home
  I. Title
  618.4   RG652
ISBN 0 09 146031 X

INCH

For Jenny

First follow nature, and your judgement
frame by her just standard.

Alexander Pope, 1688–1744

Contents

Foreword   9
Acknowledgements   12
Introduction   14

1 The evolution of midwifery   18
2 The assumption of pathology and its implications   26
3 The first stage: Alterations of the physiological
  pattern   43
4 The first stage: The active management of labour   56
5 The first stage: Pain in labour   93
6 The second stage   117
7 The third stage   145
8 Alternatives and improvements   192

Appendix 1 An outline of the process of labour   210
Appendix 2 Arranging a home birth   215
Appendix 3 Active birth   236
Appendix 4 Coping with perineal stitches: Some
practical advice   241
Appendix 5 The cascade of intervention   244
References   245
Index   271

Foreword

Many of the professionals involved in the care of women having babies believe that they are responsible for pregnancy and birth. But they see this responsibility as one that excludes the parents-to-be because birth is regarded as dangerous. The dangers, they say, are unpredictable, even given numerous antenatal examinations, and the risks can only be reduced by subjecting all expectant women to routines of investigation and treatment. Obstetricians generally also believe that only they are capable of understanding the technology required and of exercising the fine degree of objective judgement necessary to increase the safety of women and their babies.

These attitudes are, of course, contradictory. Judgement is not being exercised if all women are treated the same. Indeed, the application of routine methods of treatment gives a false sense of security and blunts the sensitivity of those applying them to the individual concerned. Thus the quality of care is often unsuitable, depriving the parents of involvement, satisfaction and the feeling of responsibility for what happens to them and their children. But worse still, I believe that this sort of care is positively harmful in that it creates disease and abnormality where it should not exist and it interferes with the establishment of the new relationships that have to grow with the arrival of a new baby.

These negative effects of modern maternity care on the experience of childbirth for parents and the children might be justified if the practices of investigation and treatment were soundly based on scientific knowledge. Most are not. New methods are introduced and routinely applied as rapidly as changing fashions in the clothes we wear. Research and evaluation of the new technology in maternity care is often poor; the results conflicting and doubtful; continued critical examination of obstetric routines is desultory and made difficult because there are few attempts to record information and results, especially with regard to the long-term future.

The assumption that lay people cannot understand the technology and the decisions involved in its application to childbearing is arrogant and wrong. This book provides evidence that people other than the professionals can understand the issues involved. Sally Inch has sifted the medical literature, and weighed and balanced the conclusions in a scholarly way. In so doing, she provides all who care to read her book with knowledge, thereby increasing their ability to understand what is happening to them. It may be hoped that such information will provide people with strength to take responsibility for themselves and enable them to question those caring for them when they feel that they have little control over events. *Birthrights*, by defining the limitations of techniques and knowledge, should help people to know when they have a right to choose. When a mother consents to a particular course of action, it should be because she understands what is required, rather than because she is coerced.

This is a very important book which will help women and men to change the attitude of the medical profession. As an obstetrician I believe that I should give back responsibility to those for whom I care and in doing so I should properly share it with them. I should provide women with choice in childbearing, thus increasing their satisfaction and sense of fulfilment in the safe delivery of their children – choice based on

a knowledge of the options available. I am grateful to Sally
Inch whose book will help me to do this.

Peter Huntingford, MD, FRCOG
Consultant Obstetrician and Gynaecologist
Maidstone Health District, 1982

Acknowledgements

I am grateful to Anne Cowie, formerly of the Cairns Library, Oxford, for her efforts in obtaining much useful research material, and to Chloe Fisher both for the drawer in her filing cabinet and for her efforts as 'runner'.

In addition to the research work actually reported (and therefore listed in the bibliography), I gratefully acknowledge the information, guidance and encouragement given to me by Dr Alistair MacLennan, Dr Murray Enkin, Nicky Lean and Sheila Kitzinger. My thanks are also due to my friends Helen and Keith Rose, who were patient sounding boards, to Eileen Frazer, Kate Newson and Jane Harrison for their help and advice, to Caradoc King for his enthusiasm and professional assistance, and to Alison Harris, who introduced him to me.

I am greatly indebted to my mother, Nora Cade, for her help and encouragement, and for painstakingly deciphering, correcting and typing the original manuscript, and to Kay Willbery for typing additional material. I am very grateful to Dr Iain Chalmers, who gave most generously of his time and expertise in reading and criticizing the whole of the original manuscript, and to Dr Martin Richards, who read and commented on the drugs section.

Special thanks are due (again) to Chloe Fisher. This book

began as a result of a meeting to which I went (in great trepidation) to speak as her last-minute stand-in. That the seeds sown there have germinated and flowered has been due primarily to her support. This has taken many forms, including the loan of books, magazines, tapes and cuttings, reading and correcting parts of the manuscript, many hours of her time, the benefit of her considerable experience, and her unfailing enthusiasm for what I have tried to do.

Finally, this book could not have been written without the help of my husband, Steve. It was through his endeavours that most of my writing time was created, and our children instructed in the delights of the Oxfordshire countryside.

Introduction

This book is written primarily for the expectant mother and is intended to take her step by step through common obstetric practices applicable to each stage of labour and delivery, and examine them critically in the light of the available medical research.

If changes are going to take place in the way in which women are treated before, during and after delivery, then the driving force must come from the 'consumer'. This was highlighted by the drop in the induction rate in 1974–5 after massive exposure in the media and consequent pressure from the relevant sector of the community, namely the expectant mothers. Attempts to change any system from within are often stifled at the outset, especially when vested interests are at stake, and the people most likely to be critical are also those who are most vulnerable in terms of their position in the hierarchy. Even when criticism comes from a higher level – for instance, an eminent professor or consultant – he is still only able to affect the policy of those directly under him in the chain of command, and can only point out to his colleagues what he is doing and why. He has no authority to make them change their practices. It is also very difficult to criticize midwifery procedures within a hospital without generating great ill feeling, even when these practices may be totally mechanical and performed without thought for the needs of an individual mother. When any process becomes part of an established routine, it becomes almost sacrilegious to ask why it is done: even to pinpoint the time when it was first advocated is quite difficult.

Not only are the findings of fellow obstetricians and paediatricians queried when they do not suit the practice of individual doctors, but in some cases even research that is actually requested to support a course of action is ignored if it happens (by accident) to prove the opposite of what was hoped for or intended.

The people who could make most effective use of the results of such research are the expectant parents. In a sense they have far more power at their disposal than the health workers, for if a particular course of action is unacceptable to them, they can simply refuse to subject themselves to it. But few people are sufficiently convinced solely by their own instincts or feelings of what is right for them that they are prepared to oppose the 'we know better' attitude of many doctors. Lack of any concrete facts to support their intuition in the face of such opposition has reduced many women in antenatal clinics to impotent fury and tears. The major function of this book is to back up their arguments with the carefully considered and published work of obstetricians, medical sociologists, paediatricians and others around the world. Interleaved with this is an appraisal of the vital role of the midwife as the guardian of normal birth, in the light of the medically inspired and government-backed move towards 100 per cent hospital delivery. This has resulted in the deliberate dismantling of the domiciliary midwifery service (thereby robbing the mother of the choice of giving birth at home) and is in fact reducing the British midwife to the position and status of the North American maternity nurse – a mere handmaiden to the obstetrician.

The midwife as an independent practitioner is at least as important for what she does *not* do as for what she *does* do during the course of a normal birth, and is equally valuable by virtue of what she prevents others from doing. In the

words of Professor Kloosterman (Chief Obstetrician of the
Wilhelmina Gasthuis, the Amsterdam teaching hospital), 'The
big danger in obstetrics is that you make physiology into
pathology, either out of jealousy (because women can make
new life – q.v. Margaret Mead) or out of idleness, or because
it is so easy to take over.' The more the midwife has been
pushed out of her role as primary caretaker of the parturient
woman, the more physiology has indeed become pathology,
and the higher are the perinatal mortality statistics. Norway,
Denmark, Holland and Sweden all rely on midwives to conduct normal labours and they have the lowest perinatal mortality rates in the world.

Much of the power to prevent the decline of the midwife
again lies in the hands of the expectant parents. They must
exercise their right to have their babies at home if they so
wish and oblige the authorities to fulfil their statutory obli-
gations (1936 Midwives Act), to provide sufficient midwives
for attendance on women confined at home in their area. In
America, where the midwife has been outlawed in most states
since 1912, vigorous attempts are now being made by the
Federal Government and by self-help groups to reinstate her.
Jean Donnison, Senior Lecturer in Social Policy, North East
London Polytechnic, in the June 1979 newsletter of the Association of Radical Midwives, writes, 'It would thus be para-
doxical if it were from America, where the fashion for active
management of parturition originated, that the impetus
should come for a return to the view that childbirth is, after
all, a natural process in which modern science has a supple-
mentary but not a dominating part to play, and that more
heed should be paid to the wishes and feelings of the mother
herself – since despite men's contribution to our understanding of it, it is still – and should be recognized to be – "women's
business".'

In organizing the material in this book it seemed logical to
start with an examination of how we came to be in our present
situation with the midwife's skills ranking a poor second to
the overall control of the still largely male medical profession,
and how with the advent of obstetric technology the science

of obstetrics has been consolidated in preference to the art of midwifery. This gives a background against which to examine various common obstetric practices in the light of research. The second section starts by questioning the assumption that all women should give birth in hospital, and then goes on to look at the possible alterations of physiological pattern once she is there, through all three stages of labour and with regard to the treatment of the newborn baby.

The third section considers some of the ways in which matters might be improved for future generations of expectant mothers, both by changing present practices and by reappraising the recruitment, training and organization of midwives in this country.

Finally, in writing this book, I do not overlook the fact that expectant parents, however well informed, still need to use tact in questioning and manipulating their attendants; and that in the final analysis they also need to be able to trust them. It is my hope in writing, that this trust will spring increasingly from mutual understanding and respect for the views of all concerned, and a continuing ability to share responsibility and to communicate throughout the conduct of the pregnancy, birth and its aftermath.

Chapter 1

The evolution of the midwife

The most usual practice, historically and cross-culturally, has been for women giving birth to be attended by female relatives or experienced female neighbours. In many communities, women who had attended several births and had thus gained experience of the wide variations in childbirth became known as midwives. Tribal customs during labour, however, were often based on superstition, magic and religious ritual – the 'science' of the time. With few exceptions, the priests and men of learning who took over the practice of medicine from the shaman or witch doctor ignored the practice of midwifery. Hippocrates (460–370 BC), who inaugurated the scientific approach to medicine, did take some part in the management of childbirth, as did Soranus of Ephesus (AD 98–138), who studied, taught and wrote a treatise on the subject, but by the third century AD men were generally excluded from attending women in labour, either by custom or by law, and the study of midwifery was ignored by physicians, so that parturient women were left largely in the hands of uneducated females. For the next eight centuries, the Church stood in the way of the development of medicine as a respectable profession, and herbs, potions and incantations were again used to heal the sick, whilst midwifery remained in the hands of superstitious and illiterate midwives. Then, in the thirteenth century, there was a revival of learning touched off by contact with the Arab world and the Islamic influence in Spain and Italy. Medical schools appeared in the universities and more and more young men of means sought medical training. But the Church imposed strict controls on the new profession, and allowed it to develop only within the terms set by Catholic doctrine: there was little taught which we would recognize as 'science'. Medical theory was largely restricted to the works of Galen, the ancient Roman physician, who stressed the idea of 'complexions' and 'humours' of man, '. . . wherefore the choleric are wrathful, the sanguine are kindly, and the melancholy are envious'. For all the Church's insistence on doctrine, accounts of medical training at that time would seem to indicate that the patient's soul was in far less jeopardy from the attentions of the unqualified and 'unapproved' practitioner than was his body from those of the medically 'trained'. . . .

This new European medical profession was exclusively male, since the universities were closed to women – even to privileged women – and licensing laws prohibited all but university-trained doctors from practising. The profession played an important role in the witch hunts of the medieval world, supporting the persecutors with 'medical' reasoning. 'Because the medieval Church, with the support of kings, princes and secular authorities, controlled medical education and practice, the Inquisition constitutes, among other things, an early instance of the "professional" repudiating the skills and interfering with the rights of the "nonprofessional" to minister to the poor.'[1]

The 'doctor' at the witch trial gave an aura of science to the whole proceedings, and was asked to make judgements about whether certain afflictions had been caused by witchcraft, and whether certain women were witches or not.

In these witch hunts, the Church explicitly legitimized the doctor's professional status, denouncing nonprofessional healing as equivalent to heresy. According to *Malleus Maleficarum* ('Hammer of Witches'), the treatise on witches published in 1484, 'If a women dare to cure without having studied, she is a witch and must die.' The witch's *methods* of healing were as great a threat to the Catholic Church as her *results*, for she relied on her experience rather than on faith and doctrine: she believed in trial and error, cause and effect, at a time when the Church was discrediting the value of the material world and had a profound distrust of the senses. By this time the 'wise woman' or witch had a host of remedies which had been tested over years of use. Many of the herbal remedies they developed still have their place in modern obstetric pharmacology. 'They used belladonna to inhibit contractions when miscarriage threatened, ergot of rye to hasten labour and alleviate the pain of incoordinate labour at a time when the Church was teaching that pain in childbirth was the Lord's just punishment for Eve's original sin. . . .'[2]

'No one does more harm to the Catholic Church than midwives,' wrote Heinrich Krämer and Jakob Sprenger in *Malleus Maleficarum.*

Despite the impetus given to learning by the invention of printing in the sixteenth century, advancement in the field of obstetrics lagged far behind that of medicine and surgery. In Germany in 1513, the first book on midwifery was printed, and was translated into English in 1540 as *The Byrth of Mankynde* and remained for 150 years the only English book on the subject, and although several manuscripts appeared during this time, they demonstrated little advance on the works of Soranus. Men were still largely excluded from the practical aspects of childbirth, and in 1522 a physician in Hamburg who dressed as a woman in order to be able to witness the birth of a baby was burned to death.

By the mid sixteenth century, attitudes were changing, and in France the celebrated surgeon, Ambroise Paré, entered the field of obstetrics. His book on anatomy, written in 1549, contained the first published reference to the use of podalic version (that is, turning the baby by the foot) for shoulder presentation, and his skill in delivering the child alive enhanced his prestige with midwives. Paré also founded a school of midwives at the Hôtel-Dieu in Paris, where Louise Bourgeois (who later became midwife to the Queen of France,

Marie de' Medici) studied. Unfortunately, with the beginnings of the maternity hospitals in France and England, puerperal sepsis began to reach epidemic proportions.

In England, after the Reformation, the Church of England
accepted responsibility for the issuing by the bishops of li-
cences for midwives. The work was practised entirely by
women, many of whom were ignorant of even elementary
facts of anatomy and physiology, as was pointed out by William Harvey (1578–1657). In 1616, a petition was made –
unsuccessfully – to James I by the midwives 'in and about the
city of London', with the support of Peter Chamberlen (the
Elder) and his brother (members of the Huguenot family who
first came to England in 1569 and for four generations practised medicine in England), 'that some order may be settled
by the State for the instruction and civil government of midwives', but proper training for midwives did not come about
until men had firmly entered the area of childbirth.

The emergence of the man-midwife, a term which entered
the English language in the early seventeenth century, seems
to have been a gradual one, and owed its impetus to the new
advances in the field of operative midwifery which had begun
in France. It is probable that Louis XIV's mistress, Louise
de la Vallière, who gave birth to a baby boy in 1663, was
delivered by a man-midwife called Boucher, who was called
in by Colbert, one of the King's closest confidants. Boucher
was probably employed in order to preserve secrecy and prevent the incident from reaching the ears of the Queen. Other
ladies of the French court also appear to have been delivered
by men, the most notable of whom was Jules Clément, who
delivered Madame de Montespan, another of Louis XIV's
mistresses, in 1669, 1670, 1677 and 1678, and the Dauphiness
in 1686 (and possibly 1682). He was so successful in practice
that Louis XIV raised him to the peerage and bestowed on
him the title of 'Accoucheur'.

French man-midwives gained vast experience as they became more fashionable and built up the school of midwifery
which attracted doctors from all over Europe.

François Mauriceau, who had studied at the Hôtel-Dieu

in 1660 and who became one of the foremost French academic obstetricians of his day, published a treatise on midwifery in 1668, and this book, translated into English in 1673 by Hugh Chamberlen, greatly assisted the progress of midwifery in Britain. In it, Mauriceau proposed (among other innovations) that women be delivered on their backs in bed – 'The best and surest [posture] is to be delivered in their *bed*, to shun the inconvenience and trouble of being carried thither afterwards . . .'[3] – instead of on the birth stool which had been in use for centuries. (The midwives in Egypt at the time of Moses' birth had been commanded to 'Kill the sons immediately, on the stools.')

In 1720 William Smellie began his career in Scotland and at about the same time Dr John Mowbray started the first school of midwifery in England, giving twice-weekly lectures. The Chair of Midwifery was created in Edinburgh in 1726. The magistrates of Edinburgh insisted upon the production of certificates from a physician or surgeon certifying that the midwife had received a course of instruction prior to practising her profession. In 1739, Smellie set up practice in London and began teaching midwifery to doctors. Over the next ten years, over one thousand doctors attended his course of lectures and clinical demonstrations, some coming from Europe and America. Despite this, in 1756 Dr John Douglas was moved to write a pamphlet deploring the state of midwifery practice in London, and suggesting proper courses of instruction for midwives, the establishment of training schools in maternity hospitals (three of which had by now been opened in London, from 1747 to 1750), and an examination before a certificate to practise was granted.

As midwifery came under the sway of the medical profession, attempts were made to curtail the practice of midwives. In 1813 the Society of Apothecaries tried, unsuccessfully, to persuade Parliament to pass a law forbidding women to practise as midwives for gain without having undergone an examination and obtained a certificate of their ability. The fact that this was not suggested primarily as a means of protecting parturient women may be seen from the maternal mortality rates at the time: mothers cared for by midwives from outdoor charities had mortality rates of less than half the national average, and considerably less than those 'achieved' by male accoucheurs. In 1872 the Obstetrical Society of London set up an examining board and awarded certificates to successful candidates testifying to their competence to attend normal confinements.

By 1886 the subject of midwifery had become compulsory for medical students and any treatment of the variations of the normal conditions, including the use of forceps, was by now firmly in the hands of the doctor.

In 1881 the Midwives Institute was set up, its main purpose being to regain status for midwives and to introduce state registration. This had already taken place in Austria, Norway, Sweden, and France during the period 1800 to 1803, and in Russia and Holland by 1865. The Midwives Institute proposed the first Midwives Bill, which was put before Parliament in 1890 but was strenuously opposed by the medical profession and failed to pass into legislation. A further seven bills were introduced between 1891 and 1900, but were all unsuccessful.

Finally, in 1902, the first English Midwives Act was passed, making state registration compulsory by law. It also gave protection to the title 'midwife' and made it a legal offence for anyone to use it who was not certified as such. It also made it illegal for any unqualified woman, habitually or for gain, to attend women in childbirth except under the direction of a doctor. The training period for registration was three months, and the Act sanctioned the setting up of the Central Midwives Board which framed the rules regulating the training and practice of midwives, and was inevitably dominated by doctors. As late as 1972, of the seventeen members of the Central Midwives Board, only four were midwives appointed by the Royal College of Midwives. In fact, until 1979 midwifery was the only profession governed by a body on which members of that profession were prohibited by law from being anything but a minority.

In America, midwives were even less fortunate. By the end

of the nineteenth century, the works of Pasteur, Semmelweis and Lister had spread through Europe and had been brought back to America by German-trained doctors who in 1893 founded the first American medical school to be modelled on the German establishments. In the next fifteen years, the practice of medicine grew from an occupation to a profession, and a jealously guarded one. With the Flexner Report (1910) behind them, and licensing laws setting the seal on the doctors' monopoly of medical practice, obstetricians in America launched their attacks on midwives: specifically, they accused the midwives of being responsible for the prevalence of puerperal sepsis and neonatal ophthalmia. Both these conditions were easily preventable by techniques well within the grasp of the least literate midwife, so that the obvious solution would have been to make the appropriate preventative techniques known and available to the mass of midwives. This is what had happened in England, Germany and most other European nations, where midwifery was being upgraded through training. Instead, under intense pressure from the medical profession, state after state in America passed laws outlawing midwifery and restricting the practice of obstetrics to doctors. The only remaining occupation for women in the area of health care in America was nursing.

With the passing of the 1902 Midwives Act in England, however, midwifery became an established independent profession. The limits of its responsibilities were set as always by doctors, but the midwife did retain the right to attend normal childbirth as a practitioner in her own right (1951 Act) with full responsibility for normal delivery. The 1936 Act had already made it compulsory for local authorities to employ sufficient midwives for attendance on women confined at home in their area. Two years later, the training provided for midwives was extended to one year for trained and two years for untrained nurses. The training period was further increased in 1981 to eighteen months for trained nurses and three years for direct-entry students.

In 1941, the Midwives Institute celebrated its sixtieth anniversary, and the title was changed to the College of Midwives:

six years later, the Royal prefix was granted. In 1951, all the midwives' Acts were consolidated into one Act (that is, those of 1902, 1918, 1926 and 1936) and just before the general election in 1979, the Nurses, Midwives and Health Visitors Act was passed, bringing midwifery into the same administrative framework as nursing. Midwives will have their own advisory committee, dominated for the first time by midwives rather than by doctors, with special provision for lay representation. At the time of writing (May 1982), this Act has still not been fully implemented.

Chapter 2

The assumption of pathology and its implications

The requirement for all women to give birth in hospital

The main argument put forward for recommending that all women have their babies in hospital is that hospital delivery is safer for all categories of women and their babies. This belief was stated unequivocally in the Peel report of 1970,[1] which became the basis for official policy in this country. Paragraph 248 stated, 'We consider that the greater safety of hospital confinement for mother and child justifies the objective of providing sufficient hospital facilities for every woman. . . .'

It did not, in fact, substantiate its assertions with any statistical evidence, but it drew attention in paragraph 29 to an increase in hospital confinements on the one hand, and a decrease in perinatal and maternal mortality on the other. There are two objections to this generalization: firstly, it is not sufficient simply to point to two trends occurring within the same time span and assume a causal connection between them, otherwise the fall in perinatal mortality could equally well be correlated with the increase in air traffic across the Atlantic! Secondly, when the data available are analysed,[2] it is apparent that not only is there no significant negative correlation between the annual hospitalization rates (in England and Wales from 1962 to 1971) and the perinatal and maternal mortality rates, but also that high mortality rates are most often associated with high rates of birth in hospital.

This was borne out by Fryer and Ashford, who analysed the effect of hospital confinement on perinatal mortality for each successive year from 1956 to 1973.[3] They found that for the first twelve years, i.e. up to 1968, local authorities with *above-average* rates of hospital confinement tended to have *below-average* rates of perinatal mortality, although the strength of this association decreased year by year. Following further rises in hospital confinements in 1968 and 1969, the trend was reversed, and local authorities with *above-average* hospitalization rates also had *above-average* perinatal mortality rates.

As has already been noted, observational data of this kind does not provide proof of a causal relationship, but it does tend to suggest that after 1967 further increases in hospital confinement rates were counter-productive in terms of producing further reductions in perinatal deaths.[4] By 1967, the hospitalization rate was 75 per cent in England and Wales, so that it would seem that a proportion of home deliveries of 25 per cent would produce at least as low a level of perinatal deaths as is currently obtained.

In the face of this, one of the arguments put forward by the advocates of 100 per cent hospital confinement is that hospital perinatal mortality rates are higher than elsewhere because a relatively greater proportion of births in hospital have more than one high-risk characteristic.

In rejecting this explanation, Tew has offered an alternative hypothesis.[5] First, turning to the survey of British births in 1970,[6] she notes that there was a very wide disparity between the perinatal mortality rate for home deliveries (4.3 per 1000 total births) and that for NHS consultant units (27.8 per 1000 total births). When the fact that there were conventional high-risk factors present in the mothers in the home group[7] is taken into account, the difference in mortality rates can only be explained if there was also an overwhelming number of risk factors in the hospital group. Secondly, by taking into account age, social class and parity (i.e. the number of babies a woman has had), one also accounts for many other 'risks' associated with childbirth, as the two sets of risks are to a degree interdependent. For example, a woman who has had a lot of children is likely to be older, *and* therefore is more likely to develop high blood pressure. Also, although the *rate* of perinatal death in babies born to women with, say, three risk characteristics is likely to be greater than in those born to women with two, the actual *numbers* affected are, according to Tew, likely to be small. Thus, it is very unlikely that the disparity in the death rates can be explained simply in terms of the number of high-risk factors in the hospital group.

A third argument that may be raised in favour of 100 per cent hospital confinement is that this would then automatically include women who had not been identified as being at increased predelivery risk, but who nevertheless make up 10 per cent of the perinatal deaths, and this would ensure a greater chance of a successful outcome. But however valid the claim may be in individual cases, the available statistical evidence does not support the assertion in general.[2] It would be misleading to suggest that death which occurred at home could necessarily have been prevented if the birth had taken place in hospital. A study of 5000 home births in Holland showed that, of the few deaths that occurred in the group, not one of these could have been prevented by hospitalization.[8]

At this point it would be useful to consider what constitutes a 'risk factor'.[9] The indications for hospital confinement have grown considerably in the last ten years, and in Holland, which still has the highest home-confinement rate in the developed world, as well as one of the lowest perinatal mortality rates, the absence of all the following indications is now a precondition for home confinement, as it is in this country.

Risk factors

1.   A woman expecting her first child (a primigravida), who is over 30 years of age.

2.   A woman expecting her second or subsequent child (a multigravida), who is over 35 years of age.

3.   A woman expecting her fourth or subsequent child (in medical parlance, para 3 or gravida 4). This is held to be a risk factor, although unpublished observations from the 1958 British Perinatal Mortality Survey show that, providing the preceding pregnancies have been uneventful, this group are not 'at risk' if they are not over 35 years of age.

4.   Low social class. In Britain a woman who falls into social class IV or V as defined by the Office of Population Censuses and Surveys. This is a very broad classification and has to be interpreted in the light of the individual woman's environment.

5.   Disorders of maternal growth – in particular women who are small or grossly overweight. A height of less than 158 cm (5 ft 2 in) is associated with a higher perinatal mortality rate. This is probably because women in lower income groups are more likely to fail to reach the full height of which they are potentially capable by virtue of an unsatisfactory diet or poor environment. The fact that the majority of perinatal deaths to women in this category are not due solely to me-chanical causes (i.e. disproportion, or the maternal pelvis being too small to allow the baby's head to pass through) supports this explanation.

6.   A woman who has rhesus problems or other forms of isoimmunization. (This does not mean all women who are rhesus negative – only those who have circulating antibodies present.)

7.   A woman who has had an operation on her uterus, e.g. a previous Caesarean section, removal of fibroids (myomec-tomy), or a previous hysterotomy to terminate a pregnancy. This again does not mean that a woman in this category cannot have a perfectly normal delivery, but simply that the presence of a scar on the uterus needs careful 'watching' during labour – if it gave way, an immediate Caesarean would be necessary.

8.   Previous third-stage problems. A history of a retained placenta or a postpartum haemorrhage (bleeding after the birth of a baby resulting in a blood loss of 1–1½ or more pints) are both strong indications for hospital delivery, as there is a strong likelihood of recurrence even if intervening third stages have been normal.

9.   A woman with a bad obstetric history, e.g. previous forcep deliveries, premature labours, etc.

10.   Previous low birth weight babies: this includes not only babies born prematurely, but also those who failed to grow properly in the uterus ('small for dates'). Babies in this group account for 66 per cent of all perinatal deaths.

11.   Coexisting maternal illnesses: e.g. high blood pressure, renal disease, diabetes.

12.   Any woman who has received no antenatal care. Women in this category are automatically considered to be 'at risk' since none of the potential risk elements have been ruled out.

13.   Any condition which may develop during the course of the pregnancy which may move the mother into a higher risk category:

(a) Pre-eclampsia (toxaemia of pregnancy). This is normally considered to be present when two out of the three possible symptoms are present – a rise in diastolic blood pressure of more than 20 mmHg pressure above the 'booking' blood pressure, or a rise above 100 mmHg; protein in the urine (proteinuria) and fluid retention (oedema).

(b) Antepartum haemorrhage (bleeding during pregnancy from the placental site).

(c) Malpresentation. Any position of the baby other than head first, e.g. breech, shoulder, or a transverse lie; or head first with the face or the forehead lying over the cervix instead of the back or top of the head.

(d) Foetal growth retardation. This means that the uterus

is not expanding at the expected rate, or that the baby is smaller than expected for its stage of pregnancy and may prompt further investigations of placental function.

(e) Poor maternal weight gain. A weight gain of less than 9 kg (20 lb) may prompt further investigation as the 1972 US Collaborative Perinatal Study has indicated that a weight gain of 9–14 kg (20–35 lb) is the range within which there is the lowest rate of perinatal mortality and delivery of low birth weight babies.[10]

It follows from the above that the woman who is over 5 ft 2 in, under 30 years of age, having her first baby, or a woman who is over 5 ft 2 in, under 35 years of age and having her second or third baby, and in social class I, II or III, and with no medical or obstetric problems, is in a category of 'low risk', and could if she so desired be confined at home or in a general practitioner unit which is not part of a consultant maternity hospital.

There are strong arguments to be made for not confining women in this low-risk group in hospital. Firstly, there is the economic argument. An analysis of the relative cost to the National Health Service (or taxpayer), in three districts in England in 1970 (Southwest, Northwest and East Midlands), showed that home deliveries were comparable in cost to the cheapest of the hospitals in each area, and were very much lower than the most expensive.[11] Furthermore, in each district studied there was considerable surplus capacity in the domiciliary service as the number of deliveries had been run down faster than the available staff. If the staffing levels had balanced the work load, the overall cost of home deliveries would have been considerably lower. A more recent study in 1979[12] comparing the relative costs to the public sector of home and hospital confinement concluded that public sector costs are 10 per cent higher for consultant unit deliveries than for general practitioner units, which in turn are 10 per cent higher than for home deliveries. By keeping out of hospital those women who have no medical reason for being there, a great saving could be made in the total cost of maternity care. Even if only part of this saving was subsequently retained for maternity services, it would still mean that large sums of money would be available to direct towards parts of the system which are in most need of improvement, not simply in terms of improving medical facilities, but by improving the health education, nutritional standards or general life patterns of particular groups at risk in the population, such as socially underprivileged or unmarried mothers.

The National Perinatal Epidemiology Unit, based at the Radcliffe Infirmary in Oxford, has refuted suggestions made in particular by the Spastics Society that more technologically orientated medical care would significantly lower Britain's high perinatal mortality rate relative to other countries.[13] It claims that the key to reducing the figures lies in dealing with the problem of poverty in underprivileged areas or groups. Sociologist Dr Ann Oakley has suggested that antenatal care alone does not prevent disaster. 'If the mother has smoked heavily, followed an unhealthy diet or simply comes from a deprived household, it can be too late to save the baby even if the mother changes her life style.'

A further improvement might be made in the short term by diverting a proportion of the money saved into domiciliary antenatal care rather than relying on all mothers to attend centralized hospital antenatal clinics. The mothers by definition most at risk (see above) are also likely to be the ones who find it most difficult to attend clinics, through lack of transport, other children requiring their care, or simply because of lack of education and not recognizing the need for regular antenatal visits.

Secondly, when there is no medical reason for the mother to be delivered in hospital, exposing her to the hospital system may in itself be putting her at greater risk than if she were delivered at home. Marjorie Tew concludes in her review of the second report of the 1970 British births survey that the place of delivery itself should be recognized as a risk factor, and the data analysed impartially[14] as there is an unexplained excess in the perinatal death rate in hospital, equal to 16 per cent of the standardized home rate. Part of this may be accounted for by the fact that the mother is much more likely to be exposed to unnecessary intervention in hospital than she would be at home,[15] and this aspect will be examined more fully in the next section.

The increased tendency for obstetric interference in hospital

One of the features of modern medicine which can be demonstrated in several aspects of maternity care[16] is that

the techniques which are developed to provide benefits for specific groups of people gradually tend to be used for more and more people, on wider and vaguer indications (on the grounds that what is beneficial for some must be beneficial for all), to the point where people who do not require any treatment at all are being given it. As this latter group will have nothing to gain from the technique, they will be worse off if it carries any risk than they would be if left alone.

An example of the 'if it's there, use it' philosophy is the use of X-rays in late pregnancy. Despite evidence produced in the late 1950s suggesting that exposure to X-ray increased the incidence of cancer in childhood, in many hospitals X-rays are still being used just as extensively, even though the dosage may be lower,[18] and in some areas, 35 per cent of the pregnant population are exposed. 'There is very little reason to think that exposure rates as high as this can be justified in terms of medical benefits.'[17] As if to confirm this thought, Carmichael and Berry have drawn attention to one hospital where the X-ray facilities were withdrawn, requiring the transfer of patients to a nearby hospital if this technique was required. This small barrier to the full use of X-rays resulted in a drop in the number of pregnant women exposed.[18] With the tendency for antenatal care to be increasingly based in hospital, wider use is being made of a broad range of diagnostic techniques in pregnancy, including the routine use of ultrasound (scans) and there is little reason to believe that the more general use of such techniques offers substantial benefits to mothers or children.[17, 19]

Another aspect of the problem is that in the eyes of some doctors 'more' necessarily equals 'better'. . . . The Director-General of the World Health Organization, giving an inaugural lecture to the British Postgraduate Medical Federations in 1975 remarked,

It might appear that . . . some doctors . . . consider that the best health care is one where everything known to medicine is applied to every individual by the highest-trained medical scientist in the most specialized institution. . . . It is frightening but expected that when a specialized group is formed to perform certain actions, it is evaluated, and continues to be supported, because of the *number* of such actions which it does rather than whether a problem is solved.[20]

In the few instances where hospital trials have been set up to evaluate the effectiveness of such 'specialized groups' the results have tended to disprove the widely held assumption that everyone is better off in hospital.

For example, hospital coronary care units offer monitoring equipment, expert medical and nursing aid, and other advantages over home care – or so it was believed until research carried out in 1976 by Mather and colleagues[21] showed that heart-attack victims who remained at home in the care of their families and general practitioners did slightly better than those admitted to a specialized hospital unit!

Doctors who 'overtreat' expectant or parturient mothers might be forgiven if their motives for doing so were those of genuine concern for the mothers in their care. Unfortunately, in some cases there is a strong element of self-interest or self-protection in their clinical management. As O'Driscoll has remarked,[22]

There is a subtle influence in obstetrics that operates to absolve a doctor who intervenes in the course of a normal pregnancy, and that, by implication, exposes his conservative colleague to censure for inactivity when an infant is born dead. This places a premium on intervention as a form of personal insurance for the doctor, although the consequences are detrimental for some patients.

This is the philosophy behind current debate in America over the routine use of electronic foetal monitoring. Many

doctors are now concerned that they may be sued for malpractice in the event of complications if they do not routinely
attach a monitor to every mother in labour, irrespective of
whether or not it is actually indicated at the time. This anxiety
has prompted new research into the effectiveness of electronic
monitors (see page 89) but the vast majority of medical inter-
ventions remain unevaluated by randomized controlled
trials,[23] which in the final analysis would be far more ethical
in protecting the interests of patients than uncontrolled in-
novation and experiment.[24, 25]

Possibly the worst aspect of institutionalized care in labour
is that there are many professionals who have yet to master
the art of inactivity in situations where their 'help' is unnecessary. This may well be a result of a training that is
geared to the 'treatment' of the pathological: Rosengren and
de Vault noted in their study of one American hospital that

. . . a modulated kind of crisis seemed always to exist in the service.
In cases where no complications were . . . present . . . an atmosphere of general apprehension pervaded the team – particularly
during delivery. In cases with possible imminent complications, the
members of the team seemed considerably more at ease; tension
lessened and they appeared able to set about their tasks in a more
relaxed and workmanlike manner. To the students, the latter situations were those in which they were actually 'learning something'.[26]

Professor G. L. Kloosterman is emphatic in his belief that
80–90 per cent of women are perfectly capable of delivering
themselves normally, without any help. He adds, 'Spontaneous labour in a healthy woman is an event marked by a
number of processes which are so complex, so perfectly at-
tuned to each other that any interference will only detract
from their optimal character. . . .' He feels that the doctor or
midwife who is always on the lookout for pathology and eager
to interfere will much too often change physiology into pathology, '. . . either out of jealousy (because women can make
new life, q.v. Margaret Mead) or out of idleness, or because
it is so easy to take over. . . .'[27] As Peter Dunn has remarked,
'We must never forget that it takes more experience, more

judgement, and more courage, often, to stand back and do nothing.'[28]

Since all aspects of the active management of labour carry a potential risk to the mother and/or child, it is totally indefensible to apply them in the absence of medical, obstetric or pressing social indications, and since induction, acceleration and monitoring of labour are very seldom, if ever, carried out at home, the hazards of unnecessary interference are more or less confined to hospital practice. The situation is further complicated by the fact that it is often very difficult to use any technique in isolation: very often, further intervention is required to counteract the effects of the initial action – the 'cascade of intervention'.[29]

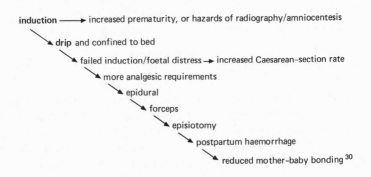

induction ⟶ increased prematurity, or hazards of radiography/amniocentesis
  drip and confined to bed
    failed induction/foetal distress ⟶ increased Caesarean-section rate
      more analgesic requirements
        epidural
          forceps
            episiotomy
              postpartum haemorrhage
                reduced mother–baby bonding [30]

(See Appendix 5, page 244, for elaboration)

Unless there is a basic change in the traditional attitude of doctors, the future is likely to bring further outbreaks of doctor-produced illness in hospitals. One way of bypassing the problem, at least for a certain proportion of the community, is to deliver low-risk mothers at home. Unnecessary interference is much less of a problem in the home setting, partly because doctors and midwives who undertake home deliveries are likely to have a noninterventionist attitude, and partly because of the technological limitations. Any act which interferes with the natural process of labour will be much more carefully considered if the machinery to correct unwanted side effects is not available. A move back to a 25–40 per cent home-delivery rate has other advantages: it would provide mothers with a degree of choice which is not yet readily available in many areas; it would allow women to develop from the moment of birth a degree of responsibility for their babies which is often denied them in hospital, and it would provide a yardstick against which the acceptability of hospital procedures to mothers could be assessed. It would moreover allow controlled studies to be carried out.

Finally, since, as has already been pointed out, hospital delivery is much more expensive than home delivery, the money that is being wasted now by providing hospital deliveries for mothers who neither want them nor need them on medical grounds could be more profitably used elsewhere.

The separation of the mother from familial support

The birth of a new baby is not an event which takes place in a vacuum: it impinges greatly on other lives, in particular those of the mother, father and existing brothers and/or sisters, and it originally took place in a home setting as part of the flow of those lives. Women who leave their homes to give birth in hospital are, wittingly or unwittingly, sacrificing a great deal in terms of their control over this important moment in their lives. In *some* cases this loss of control is certainly in exchange for the security and safety of the hospital where intervention and help is necessary; in some cases it is not in exchange for anything!

In her own home a woman is not considered a patient but an individual fulfilling a natural and highly personal task. She is the centre around which everything (and everybody) revolves. The midwife and doctor are guests in her house, and are there to assist her, and anything they do is in relation to her individual needs. This setting reinforces her self-respect and self-confidence and she retains her sense of responsibility both for herself and, when it is born, for her baby.

In hospital the reverse is true. The mother is on the territory of the doctors and midwives and under strong pressure (direct and indirect) to accept their routines and submit to their procedures. In many instances she is unknown personally to the people caring for her, and rapidly loses her individual identity as she is inserted into a broad category – 'mothers', 'elderly primips', 'grand multips', etc. She is likely to find that hospital rules bend very little to accommodate her individual wishes, and if she does not readily conform she runs the risk of being branded as a difficult patient – in some cases even to the extent of having it printed on the outside of her case notes!

It is not surprising therefore that the majority of women who have had experience of both settings and have some genuine choice elect to have their babies at home.[31] In an extensive review of current research carried out in 1964 it was concluded that the factors which affect or control uterine activity are basically the same in all mammals.[32] One of these factors is the environment in which the labour and birth take place. Ideally this should be in peaceful, undisturbed surroundings, and experiments with mice have shown that disturbances in the environment at this critical time significantly lengthen the labour and produce a much higher perinatal mortality.[33] The effect of disturbance during human labour on the human uterus is frequently seen in the admission section of hospitals as contractions seem to decrease or disappear temporarily when the mother moves from home to hospital, even if she is unafraid and recognizes her need to be in hospital. (See also page 97.) If she is not only disturbed but also frightened by her new environment, the effects on labour are much more profound, for as one obstetrician has remarked, 'there are certain conditions that predispose to normal uterine action. Almost everyone is convinced that peace of mind is important. . . .'[34] Subsequently it has been shown that fear adversely affects uterine activity and blood flow[35] and more recent investigations have linked this to changes in the baby's heart-rate patterns.[36] When the mother was exposed to a 'controlled psychic stress', her heart rate increased, and this was followed by an increase in her baby's heart rate, a condition which persisted for about ten minutes after the cessation of the stress. The researchers announced that 'in susceptible women, the entry of four or more white-coated physicians into the room is sufficient to produce changes in the heart-rate patterns of the baby.'

In many hospitals, the first thing which happens to a woman admitted in labour to a new, possibly frightening environment, is that she is separated from her husband while she is 'admitted' or 'prepared'. This often includes vaginal examinations, administration of enemas or suppositories and perineal shaving, all of which may very well be alarming or unpleasant for her, so that she might be expected to need more, rather than less, emotional support. It seems to be a feature of many hospitals that the times when the husband is likely to be asked to 'wait outside' are precisely the times when he is most needed by his wife – when examinations or obstetric manoeuvres are being carried out, progress is being assessed, and future plans are being made, among which may be the administration of drips or drugs. The main reasons for this seem to be to spare the staff the necessity of having to explain their actions before the event, or to spare them the embarrassment of carrying out procedures (such as vaginal examinations) in front of the husband! It is not uncommon for the husband to re-enter the labour room to find that his wife has consented to the administration of drugs or procedures that he knows she did not want and might have refused even in labour had he been there to back her up. In some cases also, the husband once excluded from the room is not then readmitted either because his presence is not thought desirable by the staff, or because they simply forget that he is there. Many obstetricians will not permit husbands to be present for forceps deliveries, and even fewer will allow a husband to be present for a Caesarean section. But as Dr Murray Enkin[37] points out,

The mother should have the right to have her partner with her at this important time in her life. It is true that [these are] surgical procedures, and that rigid aseptic technique in the operating room is required. But there is no reason why any intelligent man cannot be shown how to put on proper operating room attire, wear a cap and mask, and stay away from the sterile field.

Once the birth is completed, the couple, now a family (or a larger family!), are still at the mercy of hospital routine which may allow little time for them to be alone together and to get to know their new child. The baby may be routinely placed in the nursery for a specified period of time, and the husband sent out again if stitches are required. Even in the most 'permissive' of hospitals there comes a time when the husband is expected to go home, and husband and wife are thus separated at a time when they most need each other to talk to, to assimilate what has happened to them. Very often, the wife is then given sleeping tablets and the baby removed from the room, and the husband, having spread the good tidings, may be lonely and depressed as a result of spending his first nights as a father in an empty house.

For as long as the mother remains in hospital, she will continue to have dictated to her by the hospital the times she is expected to sleep, wake, eat and feed her baby. Her husband may be allowed only at certain times to visit her, and in some hospitals other children of the family may not be allowed at all. The latter is hardly likely to make for untroubled acceptance of the new baby.

The hospital continues to be 'responsible' for the baby until the mother takes him home – in some hospitals she may not carry her baby in her arms in case she drops him – and the mother is sheltered from the implications of her childbirth to the extent that when she gets home, she feels incompetent and panic-stricken, finding herself with a helpless, dependent human being to care for. Many women describe a curious feeling of having been in limbo while in hospital – a feeling that may take many weeks to overcome and which interferes with their ability to feel confident as mothers.

The degree to which the mother is regimented seems to bear little relationship to the size of the hospitals or the wards. It might be thought that in hospitals which have large wards some degree of routine was essential, but there is little difference between these and hospitals with single rooms for mothers, suggesting that the routines stem from the social organization of the whole hospital rather than from the individual requirements of the ward staff or the mothers.[38]

Very little thought is given to the effect of the hospital itself on the emotional or psychological state of the mother, or the harm that may be done to the intrafamilial relationships. One reason put forward by Dr Franklin (Consultant Paediatrician at Queen Charlotte's Hospital and Chairman of the British Association for the Study and Prevention of Child Abuse and Neglect) is that parents are always assumed to be 'normal', and capable of adjusting to their circumstances.[39] But, as he points out, 'Little attempt is made to identify those families which are vulnerable and in which the probable benefit [of routine hospital procedures] may be outweighed by the emotional and psychological damage.' He continues, 'The care of the newborn baby and the mother should be recognized as at least as much a matter of human relationships as it is of scientific method and apparatus.'

It is a fact that in a hospital setting where there is a large group of professional people with varying degrees of skills and experience, there is need for a certain amount of central direction to ensure the physical health and safety of mother and baby, and perhaps also to reduce responsibility for any sins of omission and commission. . . . If an accident occurs and the routines have been followed, the responsibility of the individual is lessened – and to some extent the mother is protected by this policy. But the price of following routines is the neglect of the need to think about the mother as an individual – indeed, one purpose of a routine procedure is precisely to spare any need to think. Yet periodic thinking about the necessity for some of the routines is essential for the comfort as well as, in some cases, the safety of the mother and child. Professionals need to ask themselves from time to time, 'Why am I doing this? Is it really necessary?' and mothers need to ask questions whenever the reason for a proposed procedure or line of action is not clear to them, rather than simply submitting to authority. If they do not feel able to do so at the time for their own benefit, then they should be encouraged to set down their complaints and questions in a letter once they have left hospital, for the benefit of future mothers. Similarly, if they were very pleased by the treatment and consideration they received, they should again say so in some form. Staff are often misled about the acceptability of hospital practices, because mothers tend to tone down their criticisms whilst in hospital, for fear of making life more difficult for themselves, and when home they then complain to relations or friends rather than to the hospital authorities. Unfortunately, in the worst of these situations where there is most need to bring to the attention of the staff the feelings of the mother for whom they are caring, the mother herself is most likely to try simply to blot out the experience and bury it in her subconscious.

There will always be mothers who need the expertise of the obstetricians and paediatricians and the machinery at their disposal, and for their sake every effort must be made to make hospital as comfortable and as welcoming as possible, given the limitations of design, staffing and organization. Mothers who do not need the 'help' which can be given them in hospitals have very much more to lose than to gain if they have no alternative but to give birth there.

Chapter 3

The first stage

Alterations of the physiological pattern

Perineal shaving

Removal of the pubic hair before delivery is a time-honoured medical custom begun at the turn of the century. De Lee (*Obstetrics for Nurses*, 1904)[1] meticulously describes the details of perineal shaving in his book and states that 'many cases of puerperal fever are due to lack of surgical preparation of the patient'. Current textbooks on obstetrics and midwifery also describe shaving in great detail and they invariably seem to accept the need without question. The theoretical advantages of the procedure are, one, surgical cleanliness is improved; two, episiotomy may be performed and repaired without hair interference; and, three, the fastidious accoucheur is not affronted. M. Myles in her *Textbook for Midwives*[2] gives shaving as the first item in her list of the details for preparation of the woman in labour. She says, 'The pubic hair is usually shaved . . . because otherwise it is difficult to keep the vulva clean throughout labour.' She also says, 'The majority of midwives prefer shaving to be done, and many think patients' objections to this have been exaggerated.' She then goes on to describe the procedure. A study carried out at Northwick Park Hospital, Middlesex, which conducts over 3000 deliveries a year, found that 98 per cent of mothers, when asked, objected to shaving.[3]

There is no physiological basis for removing pubic hair. Denman (1821),[4] Churchill (1848)[5] and Bedford (1868)[6] do not mention the subject, and all the illustrations in their books show pubic hair present. Warren (1902)[7] appears to be the first to recommend clipping the hair as well as washing with green soap but even he does not deem shaving necessary. J. W. Williams in the first three editions of his textbook (1903, 1908 and 1915)[8] suggests that 'if the pubic hairs are very long they should be cut short with scissors, or shaved'. In the fourth edition (1919) he deleted the word 'very'.

He was, however, rather puzzled by the low infection rate observed in precipitate deliveries of unprepared patients. He therefore suggested a study, which was undertaken by Johnston and Sidall, the results of which were published in 1922.[9] In 1921 Lankford[10] had described how the use of soap and water tended to wash contaminating material into the vagina, especially in women who had already borne a child, so that it seemed plausible to Johnston and Sidall to assume that the routine preparation employed in their clinic might possibly be harmful rather than beneficial. In an effort to substantiate this assumption the routine preparation was purposely omitted in 44 consecutive cases, and it was found that only 4 of them (9.1 per cent) had a raised temperature following delivery, compared with the usual finding of 19 per cent.

In view of this they decided to extend the study and in every alternate patient the routine preparation was omitted, with only clipping of the pubic hairs permitted, in a total of 389 women. Of the prepared group 16.3 per cent, compared with 12.4 per cent of the unprepared group, had raised temperatures in the days following delivery. They considered this a statistically significant difference, due probably to iatrogenic contamination. Although an additional series of observations gave identical results, Williams stated that he was not yet prepared to abandon the time-honoured method of preparation, and his fifth edition in 1924 read, 'The patient should be placed on a douche pan and the pubic hair cut short with scissors or shaved.'

Forty years later, observations similar to those of Johnston and Sidall were made by Burchell (1964) at the Research and Educational hospitals.[11] Indigent obstetric patients who entered hospital late in labour and had no vulval preparation usually had an uneventful postdelivery period. As a result of these observations a simplified method of preparation was instigated in 1960. The pubic hair of women in labour was neither cut nor shaved, but the vulva wiped with gauze to remove mucus or blood, and the area sprayed with an antiseptic. Between 1960 and 1964 more than 7600 women were prepared in this way, and the infection rate dropped.

Further work done by Kantor et al.[12] confirmed that 'shaving of the perineum in preparation for delivery does *not* permit more effective perineal sterilization.'[51] It also makes the point that 'clipping or cutting the hair round the episiotomy area is satisfactory and will avoid the irritation caused by [shaving and] the regrowth of perineal and pudendal hair.'

In spite of this weight of evidence, perineal shaving is still an integral part of the delivery preparations in many hospitals. Lomas suggests that 'there is a formality (in this and other practices) which has something of the character of a public ritual.'[13] He continues, 'We do not regard the practices surrounding childbirth in our society as ceremonial or ritualistic, but may it be that the ritual is hidden from us only because we are so hypnotized by the apparently rational assumptions behind them that we do not even begin to seek a further explanation.'

In view of all this, it does not seem unreasonable for women to voice their objections to the practice of shaving. In addition to the fact that the procedure, even in skilled hands, often results in multiple scratches and abrasions which are painful and sting when antiseptics are applied, and that the urge to scratch the irritating regrowing stubble may prove acutely distressing, there is no longer any basis for the assumption that it has any value on therapeutic or hygienic grounds.

Administration of enemas and suppositories

In many hospitals part of the admission procedure for a woman in early labour is the administration of two suppositories or an enema. A suppository is a small, bullet-shaped pessary made either of jelly or a waxlike substance, which is inserted into the rectum. Enemas come in a variety of forms, but the small disposable enema, commonly used in childbirth, is a quarter pint of a clear, watery solution of salts in a polythene bag to which is attached a small nozzle 3–4 inch long with a sealing cap. When the nozzle has been lubricated and the cap removed, the nozzle is inserted into the rectum and the contents of the bag squeezed into the lower bowel. In both cases (suppositories and enemas) the woman is required to lie on her left side with her knees drawn up, with her rectum close to the edge of the bed. After administration, she is instructed to hold the suppository or enema for as long as she can – or she may even be timed while the liquid takes effect.

Having the lower bowel evacuated in this manner is not particularly pleasant even for a woman not in labour: if she is coping with contractions at the same time, it is not only very uncomfortable but it may also on occasions be impossible for her to contain the suppositories or particularly the enema for as long as she has been instructed, or even for her to reach the lavatory in time – an event which is likely to be humiliating and distressing for her.

There are advantages to having the lower bowel empty from early on in labour: it is more comfortable for the mother, as there is more room for the baby's head to descend and rotate as labour progresses, and it ensures a 'clean field' for the actual delivery. Anything in the way of the descending head will be expelled immediately before and during the birth, which may distress the unprepared mother.

Another effect which bowel evacuation/stimulation may have is that it may stimulate the uterus. The nerve supply to bowel and uterus appears to be connected, and this feature may be made use of at the end of a pregnancy as a 'medical' form of induction. In this instance, a woman may be given a quantity of castor oil to drink, an enema and a hot bath – all in an effort to initiate labour. This procedure is only likely to be effective if labour is imminent, and a vaginal examination performed immediately prior to the administration of this oil–bath–enema procedure has revealed a soft, 'ripe' cervix. The reflex stimulation of the uterus is also the reason why an enema should not be given to a woman in strong labour, particularly if she has had a previous child, in case the augmented contractions speed labour to the extent that the baby is expelled along with the enema. For this reason also, the enema/suppository should always be preceded by a vaginal or rectal examination.

The most cogent argument against the use of *routine* enemas or suppositories is, however, that in a great number of women the physiological overture to labour is spontaneous emptying of the bowel – either as small, frequent motions or as a mild attack of diarrhoea – very often attributed to what she ate the night before! In this case, there is reflex stimulation of the bowel by the uterus as contractions begin gently. There is nothing to be gained in this very common situation by the additional administration of an enema. Even if the midwife is reluctant to take the mother's word for the fact that the bowel *is* empty, this will be easily confirmed when the vaginal or rectal examination is made to assess the state of the cervix, and it would be unkind to insist that the mother be subjected to the discomfort of an enema in this case. If there is a need for evacuants, and the mother understands the need, she is less likely to feel assaulted: if there is no need – and often there is not – the mother should not be afraid to make the fact known and thus spare herself unnecessary discomfort.

Confining the labouring woman to bed

The practice of restricting the position and mobility of a woman in labour seems to have been introduced in the first half of the eighteenth century. Until then most women in the world adopted some variation of an upright and relatively mobile theme. This might have been standing, sitting, kneeling or squatting, but always with the lower half of the trunk more vertical than horizontal. In Europe, the birth stool was a very common sight at labours and deliveries, and consisted of a low-backed chair with the centre of the seat missing, so that it was roughly horseshoe-shaped. This supported the labouring woman in an upright position without impeding the actual birth. In 1668, François Mauriceau, in his treatise on midwifery,[14] proposed that the recumbent position be adopted in preference to the use of the birth stool, a position which he advocated in order to make forceps deliveries, vaginal examinations and other obstetric manoeuvres easier, not because it might benefit mother or baby. As it became fashionable to have male accoucheurs and instrumental deliveries, so the recumbent position became widespread in Europe and across the Atlantic. By 1824, a book by a Philadelphian obstetrician, William Pott Dewees, was insisting that delivery was best achieved when the mother was lying flat on her back with her knees drawn up. The lying-in bed continued as the major determinant of posture in labour during the nineteenth and early twentieth centuries, and then, as hospital deliveries increased, it was superseded by the delivery table, and the woman lay in the lithotomy position for the birth (flat on her back with her feet in stirrups). This is now the most common position in the modern Western hospitals of the world.

There were, however, some obstetricians who were not in favour of this departure. In 1816 Merriman, also of Philadelphia, wrote, 'The patient may be allowed to sit, stand, kneel, or walk out as her inclinations prompt her; if fatigued she should repose occasionally on a bed or couch, but it is not expedient during the first stage . . . that she should remain for very long at a time in a recumbent posture.'[15]

Half a century later, Professor G. J. Engelmann in his book, *Labour Among Primitive Peoples*,[16] was writing,

A vast and important fund of knowledge may be derived from a study of the various positions occupied by women of different peoples in their labours. . . . The recumbent position is rarely assumed among those people who live naturally . . . and have escaped the influence of civilization and modern obstetrics. . . . According to their build, to the shape of their pelvis, they stand, squat, kneel or lie on their belly; so also they vary their position in various stages of labour according to the position of the child's head in the pelvis. . . . I deem it a great mistake that we should follow custom or fashion so completely, to the exclusion of reason and instinct, in a mechanical act which so nearly concerns our animal nature . . . instinct will guide the woman more correctly than the varying custom of the times.

In 1894 another obstetric text (Lusk) warned that 'the patient should be encouraged not to take to bed at the onset of labour. In the upright or sitting posture gravity aids in the fixation of the head and promotes passive hyperaemia [increased blood flow] and dilatation of the cervix.'[17]

In Britain, William Smellie had pointed out over a century earlier that the uterus contracted less efficiently in the dorsal position, and his work was still being quoted in 1876.[18] Yet, despite all this, the practice of confining the labouring woman to bed has continued to be the accepted procedure for the advantage it confers on the midwife/doctor.

In 1963 Scott and Kerr[19] demonstrated the effects of laying a heavily pregnant woman flat on her back. In this case, the enlarged uterus partially or totally blocks off the venous blood supply returning to the heart via one of the major vessels (the inferior vena cava). This has serious side effects in the minority of women (15 per cent) who have been unable to develop an adequate alternative system for returning the blood to the heart during the period when the uterus was enlarging. These women suffer from supine hypotension, and if laid flat sustain a marked drop in blood pressure, which in turn reduces the blood supply to the uterus and placenta, and hence the oxygen supply to the baby. In extreme cases this may result in death of mother, baby or both. The remaining 85 per cent are able to compensate for the obstruction by returning the blood through an alternative network of veins. However, if this group have epidural anaesthesia administered in labour, and are then allowed to lie flat, they will also develop supine hypotension. Apart from this consideration, the weight of evidence is not that lying down is *directly* harmful (although it may be indirectly by virtue of the increased need for interference), but that a vertical position has overwhelming advantages.

Dr Mendez-Bauer[20] demonstrated in 1976 that there is an increase of 30–40 mmHg pressure exerted by the foetal head on the cervix as a result of the effects of gravity, i.e. standing instead of lying down. This means that the effectiveness of the contractions is much greater, and hence the efficiency and rate of the dilatation of the cervix is improved, although the frequency of the contractions is the same. If the woman lies on her side, the efficiency of the contractions is improved somewhat, but the frequency decreases, so that the net improvement is not nearly as great as while standing, sitting squatting or kneeling. In order to prove the superiority of the upright position in practice, Dr Mendez-Bauer alternated the posture of his volunteers every half hour from the dorsal to the standing position. He found that there was an abrupt fall in the intensity of the contractions when the women lay down, and that the effectiveness of contractions in dilating the cervix was doubled when they stood up. The mothers also found the standing half hour much less uncomfortable/painful, and it was often very difficult to persuade them to lie down again. The mean length of labour among this study group (all first labours) was four hours, and none required drugs to relieve pain.

These findings were confirmed and elaborated in the Latin-American collaborative study[21] which represented the coordinated efforts of eleven maternity hospitals in seven countries. All the mothers included in the study were in the lowest possible category of risk, all started labour spontaneously at term, with anterior positions and intact membranes. At each hospital, 50 per cent of the randomly selected volunteers remained lying down in bed for the first stage, and the other 50 per cent chose their own position. Of all the mothers in the study, only 5 per cent elected to lie down. All the rest, i.e., 95 per cent, preferred to stand, walk or sit.

Nothing was done or given to those mothers that would affect their labours – the membranes were left intact and no drugs of any kind were given. Less than 3 per cent of the mothers in the study required pain-relieving drugs and these women were then excluded from the study.

The study showed that:

1. In 85 per cent of the labours the membranes did not rupture spontaneously until the cervix was 9 cm or more dilated, and none ruptured spontaneously before 4 cm.

2. When only the first-time mothers were considered, the median length of labour was 36 per cent shorter in the 'vertical' group than in the horizontal group. When all the mothers were considered, the vertical group were 25 per cent quicker in producing their babies than the horizontal group.

3. The fact that 95 per cent of mothers preferred to be upright when given the choice indicates that they were probably more comfortable when upright. This is confirmed by Schwarcz et al.,[22] who found that when mothers spent their time in different positions in labour, they reported less or equal pain and greater comfort in lateral, sitting and standing positions than lying down.

4. Provided that the membranes were intact there was no difference between the vertical and horizontal groups with regard to 'moulding' of the baby's head, caput (swelling of the tissue over the presenting part of the baby's head caused by pressure against the cervix during labour) or changes in the baby's heart rate, despite the increase in pressure on the baby's head brought about by gravity in the vertical group.

The study concluded that in normal, spontaneous labours the vertical position facilitates the progress of labour, shortens its duration and reduces maternal discomfort and pain.

It would seem wholly unreasonable, in the light of the evidence, to deny women in normal labour the right to choose the position(s) they find most comfortable during the first (and second) stage of labour, since this is also likely to be the most advantageous position for them in terms of their pelvic shape and the position of the baby.[23] It is no argument at all to say that it is more convenient for the midwife/doctor if the woman lies flat, particularly if by doing so she is likely to make her labour longer than it need be, and make her more likely to require pain-relieving drugs, with all their attendant hazards. In the words of the nineteenth-century obstetrician,[17] 'The physician should accustom himself to conduct labour with equal facility, no matter where the woman lies. . . .'

Withholding food and drink from the woman in labour

Withholding food and drink from the normal, undrugged woman in labour is a relatively new practice. In many cultures the labouring woman is refreshed from time to time with beverages of one kind or another, particularly herbal teas. African Hottentots, for example, feed soup to women in labour to 'strengthen' them,[24] the Manus give their labouring women a hot coconut soup to prevent bleeding.[25] An early obstetric text (Merriman, 1816) advocates the use of nutritional supplements in labour. 'She should be supplied from time to time with mild, bland nourishments in moderate quantities. Tea, coffee, gruel, barley water, milk and water, broths, etc., may safely be allowed.' Relatively recent European texts have continued to advocate oral sustenance. 'The labouring woman requires a certain amount of nourishment . . . her own appetite should be a certain guide to what she wishes to eat or drink. . . .'[26] 'Oral fluids, rich in glucose, such as sweetened tea or fruit juices should be given; one to two litres should be taken over twenty-four hours.'[27]

When a woman is pregnant the carbohydrates (starches and sugars) which she eats are converted as usual into glucose. But instead of being rapidly converted to glycogen and stored in the liver for future use, it remains for longer periods in her blood stream so that her developing baby has an easily available source of energy which can be used both for growth and storage as fat (+ glycogen). This is one of the reasons why pregnant women may have sugar in their urine, as the greater quantity of sugar in the blood means that some will spill over into the urine via the kidneys. The mother, however, does need to store some energy against her future needs, and this she does mainly by converting some of her blood's sugar into fat. A sudden demand for energy, such as happens in labour, rapidly depletes her low stores of glycogen (which can be converted straight back into glucose) and she has then to start using her fat stores as a form of energy. This, however, is a rather inefficient process, and there are by-products in addition to the release of energy. These by-products are called ketones, and can be detected in the mother's urine. (If they are present in large quantities, they can be smelled on the breath as 'pear drops'.) If ketones are allowed to build up in the blood stream unchecked, they will cause alterations in the chemistry of her blood and result in the weakening of the muscle cells. The uterus contracts less effectively and labour slows down.

If all mothers are starved during labour, as is the practice in many hospitals, then many mothers are likely to develop ketosis. Once detected, ketosis means that intravenous feeding has to be instigated, which adds to the pathological environment of the hospital birth. It also severely restricts the mobility of the mother, and limits the positions she can adopt as one arm is bandaged to a small board or splint and the needle in her arm is attached via a plastic tube to a bottle, which is suspended from a metal stand. In order to correct ketosis, this bottle need contain only glucose and water, but in many cases a chemical stimulant (to increase the frequency and intensity of the contractions) is introduced, rather than simply wait for the ketosis to be corrected.

The rationale behind the practice of starving women in labour is that should they need a general anaesthetic the danger to the mothers of inhaling stomach contents if they vomit while being anaesthetized is greatly reduced. The effects on the baby of depriving the mother of food and drink for many hours have not been sufficiently researched as yet. Obviously, where the condition of the mother or baby in pregnancy or early labour is such that a general anaesthetic for Caesarean section seems likely, it would be prudent to prepare her as any other preoperative patient by withholding food and drink. The problem arises when the practice is extended to all women, irrespective of their condition. The normal woman is more likely to be at risk from ketosis than from gastric inhalation. It would seem logical, therefore, to prevent ketosis from occurring rather than wait for it to occur and then correct it by intravenous means (since it is difficult to correct by oral means once it has developed).

In some hospitals, e.g. Birmingham Maternity Hospital, a low-residue diet is 'prescribed' for women in labour. It has the aim of providing foods which are easily absorbed, do not have long fibres (i.e. low in roughage), do not form a ball or clot in the stomach (e.g. milk or soft bread) and do not remain in the stomach for long periods (e.g. fats). The diet includes tea, sugar, fruit juice, toast, honey, marmite, plain biscuits, stewed apple, tinned peaches, pears and mandarins! This sort of food intake provides the carbohydrates necessary for a fairly rapid conversion to glucose, and appears to be compatible with an 'emergency' anaesthetic.

Pure glucose is rapidly absorbed from the stomach (despite the slowing down of gut absorption which occurs at the end of pregnancy) and is then readily available as an energy source. Tablets of glucose taken by mouth have the added benefit of cooling the mouth slightly as they dissolve, and also avoid the problem of having solids in the stomach.

It is likely that the majority of labouring women would not want to eat during labour, but most of them will require fluids of some sort, particularly as labour advances, as mouths dry rapidly when breathing is speeded up in the late first stage. Those who do eat large quantities, or have had a heavy meal before labour begins do run the risk of being sick when the rising and contracting uterus begins to push on the stomach – but this alone is not an indication to withhold food should the mother desire it. It seems illogical to pay so much attention to the mother's diet during pregnancy, in part to maintain her 'physical strength and vitality for labour'[28] and then to deprive her of any source of energy when she needs it most.

Moving the mother to a delivery room or bed

It is still a fairly widespread practice in this country to require women giving birth in hospital to move from the labour room to another room or worse, to another bed in another room, for normal delivery.

The point has already been made that labour should ideally take place in peaceful and undisturbed surroundings, and that fear and disruption may adversely affect the course of a labour. During the hours when a woman is in the first stage of labour, she has had time, hopefully, to acclimatize herself to the room she is in and to allow her body to 'settle in' to the work of dilating the cervix. The end of the first stage, the transition period, when sensations within her change from being first-stage to second-stage, is often the most difficult and stressful part of the labour. It is at this point, or shortly thereafter, that in institutions which have a separate delivery room, the woman will be moved. This process may involve great physical upheaval if the woman has to get off the bed and onto another bed or a trolley, and will also frequently bring about a change (usually a drop) in temperature as she is wheeled from one room to another. She will have to cope with the intrusion of portering staff and the conduct of a difficult part of her labour under a more public gaze, if she has to cross hospital corridors. The delivery room is very often colder than the room from which she has come, and is a new and pathological environment with which she is expected to cope whilst being greatly involved with the changing sensations inside herself. In many cases, this sudden assault on the labouring woman's senses has the effect of causing a decrease in or a disappearance of uterine contractions.

There is no reason, and certainly no evidence, which indicates that it is necessary for a woman in normal labour to give birth in a delivery room (often with operating theatre overtones), rather than a labour ward equipped with good lighting, suction, and oxygen in some form. The fact that this practice continues seems to suggest a lack of imagination on the part of the staff in the utilization of available facilities.

Chapter 4

The first stage
The active management of labour

Induction

Induction is the initiation of labour before it begins spontaneously but it is in no sense a replication of the events which
would occur given the passage of time.[1] The actual mechanisms involved in the initiation of spontaneous labour are complex and at present poorly understood, but it seems likely
that they involve factors in both the mother (uterus, placenta,
pituitary gland) and the baby (adrenal and pituitary glands),
and that these factors in the two are interwoven. Induction of
labour is a pharmacological process, which 'reflects only very
distantly the natural process' and it is therefore likely that
there is a price to pay for the disruption of the normal
physiology.

The most common methods employed to induce labour are:
amniotomy (breaking the waters); cervical stimulation (stretch
and sweep); oxytocin infusion; prostaglandin administration.
(A more conservative method of induction is discussed on
pages 46–7.)

1. *Amniotomy*   Either the forewaters or the hindwaters may
be ruptured (see page 82). In order to rupture the hindwaters

a Drew Smythe cannula has to be passed through the cervix and behind the baby's head to puncture the bag of waters in the region of the baby's neck. Either amniotomy forceps (like long thin scissors with a toothed end) or an amnihook (like a large blunt plastic crochet hook) is used to rupture the forewaters when passed through the cervix. Hindwater ruptures may be performed when the baby's head is not engaged or not fitting snugly over the cervix to avoid the possibility of the umbilical cord being prolapsed, and it is also easier to push a cannula than two fingers through an unripe (closed) cervix; but it is more likely to cause bleeding, either foetal or maternal, which may be so severe that a Caesarean section is required.[2]

Simply removing the amniotic fluid has no effect on the initiation of labour, and its effectiveness as a means of induction lies in the fact that in the absence of intact membranes, the baby's head is more likely to fit well onto the cervix and thus stimulate it. The effectiveness of this procedure is in part dependent on the state of the cervix: if the cervix is ripe or 'favourable' (soft, effacing, beginning to dilate) then labour is much more likely to become established without any other form of intervention. Where the cervix is unripe (long, hard, closed) additional intervention is much more likely.[3] This is particularly true for women having their second or subsequent babies. In 70–80 per cent of cases, amniotomy alone will initiate labour within twenty-four hours[4] but the remaining 20–30 per cent would have a high incidence of intrauterine infection. Opinions vary within the medical profession as to how this problem can be avoided. Some advocate antibiotics routinely once the membranes have been ruptured for twenty-four hours,[2] and others prefer not to wait for labour to be concluded spontaneously, but prescribe oxytocin infusion after twenty-four hours,[5] twelve to sixteen hours[6] or simultaneously.[3, 7, 8, 9] In the majority of hospitals, amniotomy is performed at the same time as an oxytocin infusion (drip) is set up, on the grounds that the induction/delivery interval is likely to be shorter,[10, 3] the liquor can be inspected for meconium staining (sometimes an indication of foetal distress) and a scalp clip can be attached to the baby's head. (It may be argued, however, that electronic foetal monitoring via a scalp clip is of doubtful benefit (see page 87) and that the colour of the amniotic fluid can be observed if required via an amnioscope, which does not necessitate breaking the waters.) The disadvantages of amniotomy during a spontaneous labour are discussed later in this book (see page 86) and they are equally valid (in some cases compounded) when amniotomy is performed in conjunction with oxytocin. In addition to this, breaking the waters before labour has started, particularly when the cervix is unripe, has been shown to be a painful procedure in as many as 20 per cent of women.[11] The only consideration which could possibly outweigh these disadvantages would be a genuine medical need for induction, and therefore social reasons for induction are not considered in this text.

2. *Cervical stimulation*   This is an integral part of induction by breaking the waters as the membranes are 'swept' off the lower segment of the uterus and the cervix is stretched by the examining fingers, but it is sometimes performed antenatally when the woman is at term and the cervix is found to be ripe, in order to precipitate contractions where the woman was about to go into labour spontaneously. It is thought to mimic events in the onset of spontaneous labour in a number of ways. It may trigger a reflex in the cervix (although the precise involvement of the nervous system in the control of uterine activity is unknown); it can and does lead to a release of oxytocin from the maternal pituitary gland, although this is short-lived and its functional significance is doubtful; and thirdly, it may lead to a release of prostaglandins in the area of the cervix and lower uterus, which would have a more persistent effect.[1]

3. *Oxytocin infusion*   The use of oxytocin as a means of inducing labour bears little relation to the part which oxytocin plays in initiating spontaneous labour. There is no evidence to suggest that there is an increase in the levels of oxytocin in

the woman's blood stream prior to the onset of labour, and when oxytocin is released from the maternal pituitary gland *during* labour it is in very small quantities – 2–8 microunits per minute (no greater than the minimum rate of infusion used for induction) and in spurts throughout labour, increasing in frequency as labour progresses, rather than continuously. Oxytocin, in the form of pituitary extract, has been used in the past by means of intramuscular injections, by tablets to be sucked, or given nasally. The dose when given in any of these ways was difficult to 'recover' and overdosage was not uncommon, producing spasm of the uterus and foetal distress as the major complications. Oxytocin itself was synthesized in 1953 and became commercially available two years later as Syntocinon. It was used intravenously in very low doses in the beginning and although there was little risk of overstimulation of the uterus, there was a risk of 'water intoxication' due to the large quantities of fluid which had to be transfused in order to obtain the required effect, and the failure rate was high (40–50 per cent) though slightly lower when amniotomy was performed simultaneously.[11]

In response to this situation, the concept of oxytocin titration was developed in the sixties. Instead of having the dextrose solution containing the Syntocinon 'fed' directly to the mother, with the drips per minute counted by the midwife or by a drip-counting machine (e.g. IVAC or Tekmar), the polythene tube from the infusion bottle was passed through a machine called a Cardiff pump, which caused the dose to be doubled every twelve and a half minutes, until the desired contraction rate was reached. The desired contraction rate is preset, and information about the strength and frequency of contractions is conveyed via a catheter (a thin polythene tube) which is introduced into the uterus and, having ruptured the membranes, fills with amniotic fluid. When the uterus contracts, the intrauterine pressure rises, and this rise is transmitted via the fluid-filled catheter to the pump. The pump then maintains the dose at the level which produces the desired contraction rate (plateau state). This method of administering oxytocin virtually eliminated 'failure of induction', and reduced both the induction/delivery interval and the incidence of infection; but once obstetricians had an efficient means of induction at their disposal, the induction rate started to rise. Oxytocin administration has subsequently been further refined by the development of the MM2 machine (a Pye prototype in 1979): the oxytocin is still given intravenously, via a pump, and the intrauterine pressure is still measured via a fluid-filled catheter which necessitates rupture of the membranes (although an air-filled balloon linked to the pressure recorder (transducer) is currently being developed). The MM2 uses Syntocinon in a very concentrated form, so that very small volumes of fluid can be used, and has a much slower rate of increase than the Cardiff pump (dose doubled every thirty minutes). It is programmed to respond to any increase in intrauterine pressure above 18 mmHg, which is considered to be the resting or muscle-tone pressure exerted on the amniotic fluid. The machine has a positive/negative feedback system, and can respond to the presence or absence of contractions by increasing or decreasing the dose of Syntocinon (it does not 'plateau' the dose). Once the desired contraction rate has been reached it goes into reverse and begins a gradual decrease of the dose. If the contractions also decrease, the dose rate goes back up again; if they do not, the dose rate continues to reduce. It thus makes use of the fact that the requirements for oxytocin during an induced labour vary. There appears to be a point at which the sensitivity of the uterine muscle increases, probably due to the release of prostaglandins (usually at 5+ cm). This has the effect of maintaining the length, strength and rate of contractions despite a gradual decrease in the amount of Syntocinon administered, and in some cases the MM2 can reduce the dose to the absolute minimum as normal labour supervenes.

Many of the hazards of induction are associated with the use of oxytocin, and these will be discussed separately.

4. *Prostaglandin administration* The discovery, isolation and synthesis of the various types of prostaglandin aroused great interest in the 1970s because of their effect on the pregnant

uterus and cervix.[13] Prostaglandins are not hormones, that is, not substances produced at one site and conveyed via the bloodstream to their site of action. With one or two exceptions they are locally produced, locally acting 'cell messengers'.[1] Thus, oral and intravenous administration cannot in any sense be regarded as physiological. Despite the success that has been obtained using prostaglandins to initiate labour, there is little evidence that they are primarily responsible for initiating spontaneous labour and their precise function is still not very well understood. They do appear to have a direct effect on the mechanical properties of cervical tissue, and possibly in the lower part of the uterus also. It is this effect which led to its being used in women for whom induction of labour was considered desirable, but who had an unfavourable (unripe) cervix, as it caused softening of the tissue and lowered the point at which it yielded to stretching, thus making amniotomy – with or without oxytocin – easier and more effective.[14, 15] It may be that this property renders it unsuitable for use as a means of induction in mothers who have previously had a Caesarean section, as the connective tissue of the uterine scar may also be softened, leading to uterine rupture in labour.[16]

Prostaglandins have been administered in a variety of ways. Intravenously they are as effective as oxytocin, but give a higher incidence of side effects such as diarrhoea and nausea.[4] Given orally, they have similar gastrointestinal side effects[17] and are not sufficiently effective in inducing labour in women having their first babies (primigravidae) to make them suitable for routine use.[18] They have been found to be moderately effective when given extra-amniotically (i.e. instilled into the uterus outside the bag of waters), but as this is an invasive technique, it carries a risk of infection and the gel which contains the prostaglandin needs sterilization and is unstable (it breaks down rapidly into a simpler form), so that frequent preparations of this gel are necessary.

More recently the use of a vaginal tablet to induce labour has been investigated. It has the advantage of being simple, effective and noninvasive. In terms of effectiveness it produces results which are superior to those obtained using oxytocin *without* amniotomy, but inferior to those obtained using oxytocin *with* amniotomy. It is preferable to both of these more invasive techniques in that the mothers do not have their mobility restricted, and seem to develop a uterine action similar to that of a normal labour,[17] and have no gastrointestinal side effects. Following the vaginal administration of 4 mg of prostaglandin PGE_2, Gordon-Wright and Elder found that 58.6 per cent of first-time mothers (primigravidae) and 81.2 per cent of mothers having their second or subsequent child (multigravidae) went into labour without further action (an average of about 70 per cent). Of the 30 per cent that remained, 16 per cent showed a significant change in the state of the cervix, following the use of PGE_2,[17] and thus was associated with a reduction in the incidence of Caesarean section and foetal distress when labour was subsequently induced using oxytocin and amniotomy.[15]

Disadvantages to the mother of an induced labour

The disadvantages of amniotomy have already been discussed, and prostaglandins have not been in use long enough for their disadvantages (other than the obvious gastrointestinal ones) to have come to light, so the following section will be more or less confined to the side effects of oxytocin.

'Not all the complications which follow induction of labour are necessarily due to the induction itself; some are related to the abnormality which indicated the need for induction in the first place.'[4] While this may be true when inductions for which there are strong medical indications are considered, the case becomes harder to argue when the 'indications' are widened to include those mothers with less well-defined needs, and impossible to sustain when spontaneous labours and their outcomes are compared with a matched, induced group in whom there are *no* medical or obstetric abnormalities (such a study has recently been carried out in Oxford).[19]

In order to induce a labour with oxytocin, an intravenous infusion (drip) has to be set up. This automatically restricts the movements and mobility of the mother, as she cannot put any weight on the arm with the drip, and will therefore have difficulty in changing her position, particularly when labour is advanced, and walking about (assuming that she is allowed to do so) will be harder if she has to push a drip stand about with her. With few exceptions, the wheels on a drip stand are rather like those on a supermarket trolley: they bind when they are subjected to even minor changes of direction.)

If the mother has her labour induced, there is an increased chance that she will be monitored (normally by applying a scalp clip to the baby's head and an external pressure gauge to the top of the mother's abdomen by means of a belt), as opposed to having the baby's heart rate checked every fifteen minutes using a foetal stethoscope. This procedure appears to be a feature of induction itself and not of the indications for induction.[19] These women are therefore subjected to all the disadvantages associated with monitoring (see page 88–9) which cannot be offset by even the theoretical advantage which monitoring has been thought to confer. They are therefore at increased risk of developing foetal distress in labour as a result of both amniotomy and the restricted positions for labour (see pages 85–6 and 49).

The type and pattern of labour contractions produced by oxytocin are very different from those experienced by women in spontaneous labour. In the majority of cases, established labour (strong rhythmical regular contractions accompanied by dilation of the cervix) is preceded by intermittent bouts of regular contractions, sometimes for several hours, in the days or weeks beforehand. Thus, when the true labour contractions begin, the woman may mentally dismiss them (or at least not give herself over to them entirely for some time) until she is sure that this is the 'real thing'. All of which means that she has a long period in which to adjust psychologically and physically to the stress of labour. This is not the case when labour is induced: frequent contractions start almost from scratch at close, regular intervals (3–5 minutes) and the infusion rate will be increased quite quickly (relative to a spontaneous labour) until contractions are at the level desired by the obstetrician – that is, every 2–3 minutes. The mother therefore not only has a greatly reduced period in which to acclimatize herself to contractions, but also has to cope with them at very frequent intervals virtually from the beginning of her labour.

In many cases where labour is of spontaneous onset, by the time the contractions are as frequent as 2–3 minutes, the mother is well into her total duration of labour. Moreover, the contractions in an induced labour are of a different quality from those of a spontaneous labour (they have been described as 'sharp' or 'spiteful' by some mothers). This is not surprising when one considers that the pharmaceutical levels of oxytocin in the mother's blood stream are two to four times as high as those found in spontaneous labour, but since the quality of contractions is not a factor which can be measured externally, it is therefore either not considered or is dismissed as 'subjective' by many professionals. It has been established for some time that there is an increased need for and use of pharmaceutical pain relief (pethidine and epidurals in particular) associated with induction of labour using oxytocin, particularly when the membranes are ruptured,[15, 20] and this cannot be attributed to the 'reasons' for the induction but rather to the procedure of induction itself. This is confirmed by the Oxford study[19] which found that 94 per cent of mothers having induced labours required some form of analgesia, while only 68.5 per cent of the spontaneous group needed drugs. These two groups were further subdivided and it was revealed that 49 per cent of the induced group had epidural anaesthesia, while only 13.5 per cent of the spontaneous group did. (It should be pointed out that 18 mothers (8.5 per cent) in the spontaneous onset group were 'augmented' with oxytocin during their labours, and 51 mothers (24.4 per cent) had their membranes ruptured artificially out of a total of 210.) Induction also had a marked effect on the method of delivery.

The increase in forceps deliveries and Caesarean sections has been noted by a number of observers.[19, 21, 22, 23] In some cases this is due to the type of analgesia used (forceps rates in women with effective epidurals are much higher than in those without)[23, 24] and in some cases due to the increased incidence of foetal distress (as a result of the stronger contractions)[21, 25] and in association with the increased use of narcotics.

In the Oxford study, where there were *no* pre-existing reasons among those induced which might be expected to increase the likelihood of foetal distress, the forceps and Caesarean section rate in the induced group was nevertheless very much higher – 32.5 per cent compared with 19 per cent in the spontaneous onset group. Furthermore, the excess in the number of operative deliveries in the induced group could not be accounted for by the pain relief and monitoring they received. (Forceps deliveries in the induced group were also more difficult than in the spontaneous group, for instance requiring rotation or moderate to strong traction. This may be explained in part by the higher incidence of epidural anaesthesia.)[24] They concluded that 'membership of the induced group itself appears to carry an added risk of an operative delivery' – anything other than a spontaneous delivery, but not necessarily a Caesarean section.

Another hazard of induction which is not related to the type of delivery[26] is the increased tendency to postpartum haemorrhage (PPH), i.e. a blood loss of 500 ml/1 pint or more. Brindsen and Clarke (1978) found that the PPH rate amongst first-time mothers who had induced labours was almost twice that of those with spontaneous labours. This supported earlier work that had shown[27] an 'induced' PPH rate of 8.3 per cent compared with an overall rate of 3.4 per cent for the same period. In the Oxford study,[19] the PPH rate was 8 per cent in the induced group and 3 per cent among the spontaneous-onset group. (This is compatible with the figures for the whole hospital in the preceding year in which the PPH rate for induced labours was 10 per cent and the PPH rate for all labours was 5 per cent.)[28] One possible explanation of this increased PPH is that the uterus in an induced labour is exposed to quite high doses of oxytocin for a long period and will therefore respond poorly to an intramuscular or intravenous injection of the same or similar oxytocic drug in the third stage of labour[26] and presumably responds equally poorly in some cases to the physiological oxytocin produced after the baby is born.

Disadvantages to the baby of an induced labour

The increase in the number of Caesarean sections and forceps deliveries in recent years may be in part due to the increased diagnosis of foetal distress in labour. Foetal distress was shown to increase rapidly in the Cardiff study[29] from 8.9 per cent to 20 per cent in the years 1967–73, and over the same period the induction rate (using amniotomy and oxytocin) rose from 3.8 per cent to 23.2 per cent. Although cause and effect cannot be automatically assumed,[31] there have been other studies which have shown an association between foetal distress and the use of oxytocin.[6, 30]

Liston and Campbell (1974) showed that 'those [labours] with oxytocin clearly have a higher incidence of foetal distress than those with none',[25] although they pointed out that this might be explained in part by the underlying reason for the induction. Other researchers quoted in their paper (Turnbull and Anderson, 1968; Beasley and Kurjak, 1972) have also noted an increase in foetal distress in labours where oxytocin is used. Caldeyro-Barcia (addressing the March 1974 conference of the American Foundation for Maternal and Child Health) stated in his conclusion that 'in oxytocic-induced labours . . . almost 75 per cent of the mothers' uterine contractions were shown . . . to result in a reduction of oxygen to the baby's brain'.[32] The Oxford study[19] found a slightly higher incidence of heart-rate changes in babies whose mothers had labour induced than in those whose mothers had had spontaneous onset of labour (though they did not think it significant in the statistical sense). It is possible to speculate that the increase might have been greater, relative to the spontaneous-onset group, had the spontaneous-onset group not included mothers whose membranes were ruptured artificially, and/or who were given oxytocin to accelerate labour.

Possibly more important than whether a baby is 'diagnosed' to have foetal distress in labour is the condition of that baby when born. The number of babies suffering from 'respiratory depression' – that is, taking more time than three minutes to the onset of regular respiration – is three times as great where labour is 'complicated' by the use of oxytocin and amniotomy than when labour is spontaneous. Some babies will respond to the simple administration of oxygen via a face mask; others (where respiratory distress is due to the drugs, e.g. pethidine, administered to the mother in labour) will respond to the pethidine antidote, and those who respond to neither have to be intubated, that is, have a small plastic tube put down the windpipe so that oxygen can be introduced directly into the lungs. The Oxford study had almost four times as many babies requiring intubation in the induced group than in the spontaneous-onset group, and since in this study *no* inductions were performed for medical or obstetric abnormalities, none of this increase can be attributed to the underlying 'indications' for induction.[19]

When a baby is born, its condition is rapidly assessed by the doctor or midwife, according to an Apgar scoring system. In this system the baby is marked out of 2 for each of five characteristics, thus:

	Sign	*0 Points*	*1 Point*	*2 Points*
A	Skin colour	Generalized purply-blue or white	Pink, with purply-blue extremities	Pink all over
B	Muscle tone	Limp/floppy	Moves limbs	Moves vigorously
C	Breathing attempts	Does not breathe at all	Gasps	Breathes well
D	Heartbeat	Absent	Less than 100 beats per minute	More than 100 beats per minute
E	Response to a stimulus – e.g. touch, pinprick, etc.	No response	Little response	Vigorous response

The maximum possible score for a healthy, vigorous baby is 10/10.

A baby that does not breathe will get 0/2 in Section C and if it does not breathe, its colour will be poor, either 0/2 or 1/2 in Section A. If this situation persists without treatment, its condition will deteriorate (heart rate will start to slow, blueish colour will become more pronounced) and its original maximum score of 7/10 will start to drop. The Cardiff study showed an 'apparent increase [in the number of babies born with an Apgar score of between 4 and 7] from 13.8 in 1967 to 22.2 in 1973, during which time the number of labours induced with amniotomy and oxytocin also rose, from 3.8 per cent in 1967 to 23.2 per cent in 1973'. Again, one cannot automatically assume that the two factors are directly related, but it seems reasonable to suggest that the rise in induction may have played some part in the rise in the number of hypoxic babies.

One of the ways in which induction and hypoxia at birth may be connected is the increased use of drugs in labour.[15, 19, 20] Most of these have the effect of depressing the baby's breathing at birth,[33, 34, 35] and/or its Apgar score.[36] Richards concludes[37] that there is little doubt that the combination of greater use of analgesic drugs and the more violent contractions of the accelerated labour can produce depressed babies.

Another factor which will contribute to the increase in respiratory depression is the relative immaturity of induced babies. If induction of labour is performed before term, the baby's lungs are more likely to be unready for use outside the womb. Normally, the mature baby's lungs require an initial effort to inflate them, but thereafter the surface tension in the lungs is high enough to prevent them from collapsing right down again when the baby breathes out. When this is not the case, the baby suffers from respiratory distress and each breath requires the same effort as the first one. This is still a significant cause of perinatal deaths. Sometimes, the 'age' of the baby in utero is incorrectly assessed, and the infant produced as a result of the induction may be so immature as to develop foetal distress. (One of the babies in the Oxford study which developed respiratory distress was thought at induction to be of 39 weeks' gestation, and was subsequently assessed at 36 weeks' gestation.)[19]

Jaundice in babies has also become much more common in recent years. The precise reasons for this are uncertain but it has been shown to be associated with the use of oxytocin for induction and acceleration.[38] Martin and colleagues in Ireland have also published work which is highly suggestive of a causal relationship which may even be dose-dependent.[28] The increase in the use of forceps for delivery (as a result of the increased use of epidurals) has also been shown to relate to the rise in the incidence of jaundice,[39] and it may be that one of the factors increasing the jaundice rate is the amount of bruising the baby receives at delivery.[40]

In many cases, jaundice in babies a few days old requires no treatment, but if it is severe and a blood test shows that the levels of bilirubin (the substance which gives the skin its yellow colour) are very high, the baby may need to be admitted to a special care unit for phototherapy (treatment under lights). If it is even more serious, exchange blood transfusions may be undertaken. Many of the factors discussed above – forceps or Caesarean delivery, respiratory depression, foetal distress, respiratory distress syndrome – may all result in the baby's needing treatment in a special care unit. With very few exceptions this means that the mother and baby have to be separated and it is now well established that separating mother and baby at birth may have important consequences (see also page 184).

Having considered the means and the possible hazards of induction, one ought to look at the possible benefits. Social considerations apart, an induction is medically justifiable only when the risks inherent in the procedure are less than those which could be expected were the pregnancy allowed to continue: to put it another way, only when the danger to the mother and baby, if the latter remains in utero, are greater than those of induction and delivery.

There are some obstetric conditions in which it may be hazardous for the pregnancy to continue to term, and in these cases preterm delivery may prove valuable. In a high proportion of these cases, however, this may indicate an elective Caesarean section rather than induction of labour, as the stress of labour on top of an already compromised foetal blood/ oxygen supply may precipitate acute foetal distress.[41] Conditions which might be included in this category are: rhesus isoimmunization, essential hypertension, renal disease, pre-eclampsia with proteinuria (i.e. protein present in the urine) and diabetes.

1. *Essential hypertension* (occurs in 1–3 per cent of pregnancies)[41] This is a sustained rise in blood pressure prior to pregnancy which is precipitated by a generalized spasm of the smaller arteries (arterioles) which in turn leads to a greater resistance being offered to the flow of blood. The reason for this is unknown, but the effect is to reduce the blood supply to the uterus, and as a consequence the formation of the placenta may be affected and the foetus may fail to grow properly. If the hypertension is severe, the mother's health may also be affected. In about 30 per cent of cases, protein appears in the urine, so that the condition is indistinguishable from severe pre-eclampsia.

2. *Renal disease* (occurs in 0.2 per cent of pregnancies)[41] Well-controlled renal disease (glomerular nephritis) which has occurred before the onset of pregnancy will only complicate a pregnancy if it is accompanied by a significant rise in blood pressure – which happens in about 40 per cent of cases. In these circumstances, the situation is similar to that in (1) above, in that reduced placental blood flow may affect foetal growth. If the actual function of the kidneys has been affected by the disease, i.e. the ability of the kidneys to

filter off and excrete toxic waste, the foetus is relatively unlikely to survive (60 per cent die in utero)[41] and the mother's health may be seriously affected.

3. *Pre-eclampsia* (occurs in 6 per cent of all pregnancies – 12 per cent of first pregnancies) This is considered to be severe when there is more than a trace of protein in the urine and the diastolic blood pressure – the bottom reading – is over 100 mmHg. It does not normally occur before 28 weeks of pregnancy, so the placenta is likely to be normally formed. Severe pre-eclampsia is associated with a reduced blood supply to and reduced function of the placenta. In addition, the mother's other organs may be affected when visual, gastric or cerebral disturbances are present. Pre-eclampsia is usually a slowly progressive disorder, but it may suddenly develop or suddenly become severe, and the mother's health deteriorate. In these cases, termination of pregnancy by Caesarean section is indicated, whatever the duration of pregnancy. About a quarter of mothers with severe pre-eclampsia are suitable for induction rather than Caesarean section, but O'Driscoll and colleagues have suggested that 'a conflict of purpose is introduced . . . every time a foetus who is considered to be at risk is subjected to an extended period of stress with oxytocin'. It should be emphasized that the overall incidence of these three conditions is only about 8 per cent of the pregnant population, and in only a small proportion of these is induction preferable to Caesarean section in order to produce a live baby.[41]

4. *Rhesus disease or isoimmunization* It is difficult to estimate the precise incidence of the disease as opposed to the mortality,[42] but in 1969 it was estimated to occur in 0.5 per cent of pregnancies,[41] and this figure is probably very much lower now.

The problem occurs in a rhesus negative mother who carries a rhesus-positive baby. In normal circumstances, it is of no consequence in the first pregnancy unless the mother has received rhesus-positive blood from some source prior to the first established pregnancy, as happens in a very few instances. This could occur with a blood transfusion, or a miscarriage/abortion where there was no medical supervision (and therefore no anti-D was given). When the first birth takes place, some placental (foetal) blood may escape from the placenta into the maternal blood as the placenta separates. If nothing is done about it, the mother's body will react (over the next 60 hours) to the presence of this foreign material and produce antibodies which will destroy it. These antibodies will remain present in the mother's blood stream and are small enough to cross the placenta in a subsequent pregnancy, when they will begin to destroy the baby's blood cells.

There are several reasons why this condition is not as frequent as formerly: these include changes in the birth rank (i.e. fewer women have large numbers of children), and as the disease is worse in successive pregnancies the reduction in the number of births per woman will reduce the overall incidence of the problem and its severity; general improvements in perinatal and obstetric care, and the introduction of high potency anti-D gamma globulin (1gG) which when administered within 60 hours of delivery to a rhesus-negative mother, will prevent the formation of antibodies.[43] All this means that the use of induction to terminate a pregnancy in which rhesus disease is severe after 34 weeks (before that, Caesarean section is preferred)[41] will affect only a very small proportion of women.

5. *Diabetes* (between 0.1 per cent and 0.3 per cent of women of childbearing age are diabetic)[41]   The main problems associated with pregnancy in a diabetic woman manifest themselves after the 28th week, when the incidence of pre-eclampsia and polyhydramnios (too much amniotic fluid) increase, and the perinatal mortality rises rapidly after 38 weeks. Most of the deaths occur in the uterus, some in labour and some in the newborn period, usually of respiratory distress syndrome. The cause of death is unknown, but it is thought

to be due to altered exchange mechanisms in the placenta.[44] (Congenital abnormalities are also thought to be higher in diabetic pregnancies.) Because there is a rise in the perinatal mortality after 38 weeks' gestation, the baby is usually delivered during the 37th week: this will necessarily result in a premature baby, and the mortality in premature babies is already higher. (In some units, however, where there is excellent control of diabetes babies are now delivered at 40 weeks.) Part of the raised perinatal mortality rate associated with diabetes also stems from the premature labour brought about both by the increased size of the baby when diabetes is poorly controlled, and by polyhydramnios, both of which 'stretch' the uterus.

Caesarean section is the usual method of delivery (when there are no known abnormalities which would be incompatible with life, and the baby is alive). Induction of labour in selected diabetic primiparous and multiparous women with a history of previous uncomplicated deliveries has its advocates, but it is thought to increase the perinatal mortality rate.

Induction and placental insufficiency

A pilot study conducted by O'Driscoll and colleagues in Ireland[45] came to the conclusion that induction was seldom undertaken in the interests of the mother, and that the indications entered in the records could often not be substantiated in the interests of the child. They also stated that almost the only foetal indication for induction of labour was 'placental insufficiency', and that this could occur as a primary condition without any maternal abnormality. Placental insufficiency is a blanket term – usually what is meant is that the placenta is normally formed and functioning in the early stages of pregnancy, but that then something intervenes to impair the function of the placenta. The condition is usually diagnosed in retrospect when the uterus does not enlarge as quickly as expected, or when a baby is delivered smaller than expected for the period of gestation, and the term 'intrauterine growth retardation' is used. Sometimes the underlying cause is apparent (see 1–4 above), but often it is not. Sometimes, intrauterine growth retardation is detected during pregnancy, both clinically and biochemically, and sometimes it is not apparent until after the baby is born.

Placental insufficiency also refers to a form of placental failure, as the oxygen need of the baby exceeds that which can be supplied by the placenta. Since this is a feature of later pregnancy, it does not manifest itself as intrauterine growth retardation: sometimes the cause is apparent, e.g. partial separation of the placenta which is usually accompanied by a small bleed (antepartum haemorrhage) but which is not so great as to cause immediate foetal death or to warrant immediate intervention. Very often, however, it is not apparent, and it is deaths in this category which are referred to as 'mature – cause unknown'. These are the deaths which many obstetricians consider preventable and which have been given as the reason for introducing high rates of induction.[46] Where perinatal mortality has been reduced, it is often ascribed to the beneficial effect of a liberal induction policy. One of the difficulties in the prevention of the 'unknown-cause' deaths is precisely that their cause is not known, and since other factors were changing during the period when the induction rate was rising, it is equally plausible to attribute the fall in deaths to obstetric and paediatric influences other than induction.[47] The study that took place in Glasgow in 1977 (McNay and colleagues)[46] is often quoted by advocates of an aggressive approach to induction of labour, as it concluded that 'the increased use of induction for labour has contributed to an improved perinatal mortality rate'. There have been several objections to this conclusion from other quarters; it was pointed out by Leeson and Smith[44] that over the period in question there had been a general falling tendency in perinatal mortality rates for most parts of the country, and that in Glasgow the increasing rate of induction actually interrupted the general downward trend during the early years (the induction rate began to increase after 1970, and in 1970, 1971 and 1972, the perinatal mortality was higher than in 1969). Furthermore, they drew attention to the fact that no comparison had been made between the perinatal mortality rate of an induced group and the perinatal mortality rate of a non-induced group over the same period.

Other observers showed surprise that the authors of the study had failed to comment on the fact that the 'mature unknown' death rate failed to improve as the induction rate rose between 1974 and 1975.[47] In total contradiction to the findings in Glasgow, another large maternity hospital with over 7500 deliveries per year showed that the perinatal mortality rate *decreased* from 38.4 to 16.4 (per 1000 total births) as the induction rate *decreased* from 26.3 per cent to 10 per cent.[48]

The Cardiff study which analysed the trends in management and outcome of pregnancy in nearly 40,000 deliveries to women resident in Cardiff between 1965 and 1973 revealed no striking change in either the total perinatal deaths rate or the timing and cause of perinatal deaths.[29, 49] Further work in Cardiff compared the work and results of two obstetric teams with contrasting liberal and conservative policies in the same city over a five-year period. It failed to demonstrate that any significant advantage was conferred by the wider use of induction.[50]

Intrauterine growth retardation is not always easy to pinpoint. Sometimes the tests used to assess the state of the placenta, either directly or indirectly, identify cases where none exists, e.g. out of 289 predicted cases of foetal growth retardation reported by M. Hall and colleagues only 83 actual cases materialized,[51] and in many cases growth retardation is not picked up where it *does* exist, for out of the 5 perinatal deaths which occurred in the pregnancies studied by O'Driscoll *et al.*, 4 were due to foetal growth retardation (all the babies weighed much less than expected for the gestation time) and the decision to deliver these babies could have been made only on an individual diagnosis of intrauterine growth – even a 'liberal' induction policy would not have induced these particular cases.[45] Furthermore, two of the tests currently used to detect either placental insufficiency or the effects of placental insufficiency, namely urinary oestrogen assay ('oestriol collections') and serial ultrasound cephalometry (scans), were not associated with any differences in the perinatal mortality rates in the comparison study in Cardiff,[50] or in the work published by Beard.[52] One study has shown that the number of foetal movements felt by the mother in a 12–hour period is a better indication of foetal well-being than 24-hour urinary oestrogen assay. A daily foetal movement count (12 hours) of above 10 was generally associated with a good outcome, even in mothers deemed to be at risk. On the other hand, a low foetal movement count was associated with a high incidence of foetal asphyxia and intrauterine death, even when urinary oestrogen levels were normal.[53]

The concept of high risk has greatly influenced contemporary obstetrics. Although it may be the case that pre-eclampsia and prolonged pregnancy are associated with an increased perinatal mortality,[54] (due to placental insufficiency), it does not follow that placental insufficiency is a feature of all cases of pre-eclampsia or prolonged pregnancy.[45] Butler and Bonham themselves showed that perinatal deaths as a result of pre-eclampsia are increased only when the pre-eclampsia is severe, i.e. the diastolic blood pressure is above 100 mmHg and there is protein in the urine. It follows that pre-eclampsia without these two factors is seldom a valid reason for induction. Nevertheless, in many hospitals every case of pre-eclampsia is induced, no matter how slight. (The Glasgow study actually showed a slight rise in the perinatal mortality rate due to pre-eclampsia, despite their aggressive induction policy, and it is tempting to suggest that this has itself made the point referred to earlier, namely, that if the baby is at risk as a result of maternal pre-eclampsia the risk is increased when he is subjected to 'an extended period of stress with oxytocin'.[45])

Prolonged pregnancy (i.e. a pregnancy lasting more than 41 weeks, or 42 weeks by some definitions), which was shown by Butler and Bonham[54] to be associated with an increased perinatal mortality, is the most common reason given for induction.[37] In the Oxford study, over half of the inductions were performed for this reason, in the absence of any other medical or obstetric abnormalities (110 out of 210). Prolonged pregnancy is not normally associated with placental insufficiency[45] so presumably the increased incidence of foetal death and foetal distress in labour is due either to a decline in placental function or to the oxygen needs of the baby exceeding the placenta's ability to supply it – but it does not follow that this will be the case in all prolonged pregnancies. Schneider and colleagues[55] subjected 104 mothers with 'prolonged pregnancy' to weekly oxytocin challenge tests and 24-hour urine collections for oestriol measurement three times per week. An oxytocin challenge-test entails monitoring the heart rate of the baby (externally) and uterine activity in the mother for 20 minutes, and then giving a very small dose of intravenous oxytocin via a drip and increasing the dose until three uterine contractions are observed in two consecutive 10-minute periods, at which point the test is considered complete. The test is considered positive (i.e. bad) if the baby's heart rate drops at the end of a contraction on three or more consecutive occasions. Positive OCTs were registered in 7.6 per cent of cases; these were delivered immediately and thus eliminated as possible cases of foetal deaths. Prolonged pregnancy managed in this way was not associated with an increased perinatal mortality rate, but the incidence of foetal distress in labour and babies requiring resuscitation after birth was increased. (Oestriol measurements were not helpful in predicting the state of the baby, either in labour or after delivery.)

A year later in 1979, Homburg and colleagues[56] gave 97 mothers with prolonged pregnancy oxytocin challenge tests and amnioscopy (looking at the colour of the amniotic fluid behind the intact membranes by inserting an amnioscope into the vagina just through the cervix) every 48 hours. (Amnioscopy was considered positive if meconium was present in the amniotic fluid.) In the interval, 24-hour urine collections were made and foetal movements were counted. (Foetal-movement counts in this case were made by counting the number of movements in a one-hour period in the morning and a one-hour period in the evening, and expressing the results as a daily mean. In this study, a count of 15 or less was considered low.) If *both* amnioscopy and OCT were positive, the mothers were delivered immediately (usually by Caesarean section). If *either* was positive, then labour was induced by amniotomy and oxytocin. Oestriol levels and foetal movements did not influence the decision to induce labour, and were not predictive of foetal distress except when combined with other positive test results.

This method of screening was rapid, reliable and highly predictive of foetal distress. Of the 50 mothers in the study with all four tests negative, only one developed foetal distress in labour. In 24 of the remaining cases, where OCT and amniotomy were negative but either foetal movements or oestriols were abnormal, only one developed foetal distress at labour.

The study concluded that the judicious application of tests of placental function may help to reduce perinatal mortality and morbidity (e.g. foetal distress or babies needing resuscitation). They also stated that these measures would detect the cases which *needed* intervention and thus eliminate unnecessary inductions of labour. This statement was in agreement with the conclusion reached by MacLennan[57] that induction should not be performed on the basis of the patient being in an epidemiological 'at risk' group, but more specifically on the basis of abnormal foetal monitoring tests.

It will be apparent from the above that there is great controversy amongst obstetricians as to what constitutes an indication for induction, and 'the truth of the matter is that [we are all] largely ignorant about the circumstances in which the benefits of induction outweigh its disadvantages'.[58] Until more randomized controlled trials are carried out to assess the validity of some of the 'indications' for induction, simply advocating high levels of induction in the hope that it will lower perinatal mortality is a highly unscientific way to proceed, and highly unethical when it exposes very large numbers of normal mothers and babies quite unnecessarily to the risks associated with induction. It behoves those who advocate induction to demonstrate its superiority in specific situations by appropriately designed research.[58]

Acceleration

This differs from induction (which refers to the initiation of labour) in that it involves the use of oxytocin (or amniotomy) in women whose labours have already started, in order to speed them up.

Initially it was advocated to improve the efficiency of labours that were progressing slowly, to avoid the problems to mother and and baby associated with 'prolonged labour' (labour lasting more than 24 hours). Statistically speaking, prolonged labour is more likely to be a feature of first labours, particularly if the mothers are over 30 years and/or under 61 inches tall (5 ft 1 in). But even so, it is likely to affect only 5–15 per cent of first labours and 2–5 per cent of subsequent labours.[59]

The longer the duration of prolonged labour, the higher is the incidence of maternal mortality due to infection, traumatic delivery and shock, but these are very rare causes of death in developed countries where Caesarean sections are performed with relative safety. The baby is also at increased risk from infection, hypoxia (from prolonged reduction in placental circulation) and trauma from difficult delivery. The main cause of prolonged labour as determined by a study in Edinburgh in 1956[60] was inefficient uterine action (50 per cent due to the quality of the uterus, 25 per cent due to the position of the baby) and the overall incidence of prolonged labour was 3 per cent. This is a lower figure than the 5–15 per cent quoted above, because those mothers in whom there was disproportion (a pelvis too small to allow the passage of the baby's head, which would obviously cause prolonged labour) had largely been delivered by Caesarean section before they had been in labour for 24 hours. Since the use of oxytocin can affect the labour beneficially only by improving the efficiency of the uterine contractions, it would appear that it will be of use only in 2.1 per cent of the pregnant population. The prediction of those mothers in whom prolonged labour will be a problem if left untreated is obviously important. This may be done by means of a partogram, which is a graph on which cervical dilatation is measured against time. The expected rate of progress is indicated by an 'alert line' drawn on the graph, and the individual mother's progress is plotted on top of this. In some cases, the alert line is straight, assuming a rate of progress of 1-cm dilation per hour, and in some cases it curves towards the time axis, in recognition of the fact that many labours do not begin at such a fast rate.

This is illustrated by the two examples below:

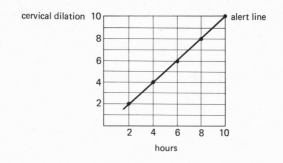

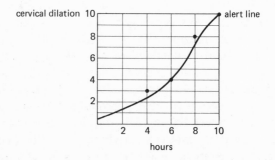

If labour is accelerated whenever it is seen to cross the alert line then not only will all mothers at risk from prolonged labour be 'speeded up', but also all those mothers in whom labour would have just taken longer than average, particularly for the first half of labour, but who are not in a category of high risk.

The 'longer-than-average' mothers, who can be distinguished from the 'prolonged' mothers only in retrospect, will have nothing to gain from the acceleration, and nothing against which to offset the potential hazards associated with the use of oxytocin. In addition, vaginal examinations will have to be made more frequently to check progress and plot an accurate time.

All the hazards associated with the use of oxytocin (with the exception of an unexpected prematurity), which have already been listed when it is used for induction, are also valid when considering acceleration, in particular the increased use of pain-relieving drugs and the associated increase in the rate of operative deliveries and delivery of 'depressed' babies.

One of the enthusiastic advocates of acceleration of labour, O'Driscoll,[61] suggests that all mothers should be educated to expect delivery within eight hours of admission to hospital by the early use of oxytocin and amniotomy when progress is deemed to be slow and labour terminated by Caesarean section if it is not completed within 12 hours. By controlling the duration of labour he maintains that the allocation of one nurse/midwife to one patient is possible, and that the need for analgesics will be reduced because the mother's exposure to stress is reduced, partly because the length of labour is potentially reduced, and partly because the approximate time of delivery can be predicted (in all but a minority of cases). He also maintains that there is an 'inverse ratio between the need for analgesia and the quality of care in the delivery unit, which is most likely to reflect the degree of personal involvement of senior medical personnel in the management of labour'.

Whilst the aims and motives expressed may be admirable, it could be argued that in the absence of medical indications for intervention, or controlled trials to prove the superiority of such a policy, the same ends could be achieved if more consideration were given to the physiological and psychological ways of preventing 'long' labours, which would of course include the provision of continuous care by one nurse/midwife and the personal involvement of the medical staff.

Amniotomy (Breaking the waters)

When the baby is developing inside the uterus during pregnancy, it does so within a double membrane. The outer membrane, called the chorion, is thin, opaque and easily torn, and the inner membrane, called the amnion, is smooth, tough and translucent. The term 'amniotomy' actually refers only to this inner membrane, but in fact both membranes are ruptured. This bag of membranes contains a variable amount of fluid (the waters) ranging from 500 ml to 1500 ml (1–3 pt). The fluid distends the 'bag' and allows the free movement and growth of the baby. It also acts as a barrier to external infection, i.e. from the vagina, and as a shock absorber, protecting the baby to a large extent from jarring and injury.

When labour starts, the fluid and membranes take on another, equally important hydrostatic function: as the uterus contracts, the pressure inside it rises, and this rise in pressure extends to the baby's circulatory system within the placenta, cord, brain, skull and scalp. At the same time, the pressure of the amniotic fluid pressing on the outside of the baby also rises. Thus, while the membranes are intact, the rise in 'water' pressure outside compensates for the rise in pressure inside the baby. It also tends to reduce the downward pressure on the baby's skull bones, particularly when the head is engaged.[62]

In view of the importance of the membranes in the normal physiology of labour and the undesirable consequences to the baby of amniotomy shown by recent research,[62] it would seem appropriate to question the common obstetric practice of rupturing the membranes artificially as a routine procedure early on in labour. This manoeuvre is unjustified in spontaneously starting labours with a low-risk baby where normal progress is being made. The commonest reason given for (midwives) breaking the waters in these circumstances is that labour will be speeded up thereby (see below) and another is that the labour needs to be monitored electronically. Foetal monitoring if indicated could be started by methods that do not involve breaking the waters. Either an external foetal electrode/transducer can be used, or else a thin catheter attached to a transducer can be inserted between the intact membranes and the uterine wall.[63]

Amniotomy could be performed later in labour if suspicious signs of foetal distress appear on the monitor tracing, such as a late fall in the baby's heart rate occurring after the contraction has passed its peak,[64] variable rhythms, or a fall in heart rate coinciding with the peak of a contraction.[65] The waters would be broken in these instances to allow a blood sample to be taken from the baby's scalp for a more accurate determination of its condition, and also possibly to insert a small electrode into the scalp.

When do the membranes rupture spontaneously?

In a recent study[66] a group of 517 mothers with 'normal' pregnancies were allowed to labour without the membranes being disturbed artificially. Of the group, 66 per cent had intact membranes at the end of the first stage. Of these, 34 per cent ruptured at 10 cm (the end of the first stage and beginning of the second), 20 per cent ruptured during the second stage, and 12 per cent still had the membranes intact at delivery. The fact that in two-thirds of the group, the membranes did not rupture until the end of the first stage suggests that late rupture is a necessary feature of the normal process of labour. Other researchers in the same collaborative study[67] found that in 85 per cent of women labouring normally the membranes did not rupture spontaneously until the cervix was 9 cm (or more), dilated, and none ruptured spontaneously before 4 cm.

What are the differences in effects of early and late rupture?

1. *Duration of labour*   When two large groups were compared – 464 with membranes ruptured between 4–5 cm, and 380 with membranes ruptured at 10 cm – and the results analysed,[68] the labours of the early-rupture group were shown to be shorter by an average of 50 minutes. This was confirmed by Dr R. Caldeyro-Barcia,[69] who found an overall reduction

of 40 minutes in the labours of the early-rupture group. The probable explanation for these findings is that when the membranes are no longer present between the head and the cervix, the head makes closer contact with the cervix and dilates it more efficiently. This is likely to be at the expense of the greater possibility of mechanical damage to the skull and underlying structures as the protection conferred by intact membranes is removed. Caldeyro-Barcia has gone so far as to say that he considers early rupture, even when it happens spontaneously, to constitute an actual complication.[70]

2. *Formation of caput succedaneum*   This is an odematous swelling on the baby's scalp due to the pressure of the cervix. The ring of pressure interferes with the venous blood supply and causes the area lying over the cervix to become congested. When caput formation has taken place it is apparent at birth, and usually disappears within 36 hours. There is a very strong association between the time that the membranes rupture, relative to delivery, and the formation of caput: from a 34 per cent incidence with early rupture down to 5 per cent with late rupture.[67]

When the membranes are not present, there is no compensatory compression of the scalp, and with each contraction, small amounts of blood and serum are squeezed out of the scalp vessels: it is this which produces the caput. Although no harmful effects can be attributed to the caput itself, it may be an indication of similar circulatory disturbances occurring within the baby's brain tissue.

3. *Disalignment of the baby's skull bones*   The pressure on the baby's head, even with a normal labour and intact membranes, is greater on the central skull bones (the parietal bones) than on the others.[71, 72] As a result, these tend to protrude in relation to the bones at the back and front (the occipital and frontal bones). This is called 'moulding', and can be considered as physiological provided that it occurs only in a minor degree.[73] However, the more marked the moulding, the greater is the likelihood of damage to the cerebral mem-

branes and blood vessels in the brain beneath. The bleeding that results when these are damaged is often severe, as the blood vessels are relatively unsupported. According to Fredric and Butler[74] the incidence of bleeding associated with the tearing of brain tissue increases according to the number of hours elapsing between rupture of the membranes and delivery. In accordance with this, the longer this interval, the greater is the incidence of mental retardation in children studied by Muller.[75] The fact that there is relatively high disalignment of the parietal bones even in babies whose mothers' membranes ruptured late suggests that membrane rupture is not the only factor involved in disalignment: nevertheless there is a strong correlation between early rupture of the membranes and the degree of bone disalignment in the baby's skull.[76, 77] This is borne out by postmortem results presented by Phillip Schwartz[78] who again emphasized the role played by rupture of the membranes as a cause of impairment of brain function.

4. *Changes in the baby's heart rate*   A transient fall in heart rate, which is synchronous with the uterine contraction that produces it (a Type I dip as shown on a foetal monitor), has been shown to have several causes: uneven compression and deformation of the baby's head during contractions (resulting in stimulation of the vagus nerve),[79] engagement of the head in the pelvis during labour, and interruption of the blood flow through the umbilical cord.[77] A study carried out to investigate the relationship between the state of the membranes, the engagement of the head and changes in heart rate[63] concluded that the incidence of changes in heart rate (Type I dips) was lower when the membranes were intact, both before and after the head had engaged. There was an even greater difference in the two rates *after* the head was engaged: i.e. much lower in the intact group.[80]

Marked changes in heart rate have also been shown to occur in a proportion of babies who have a loop of cord round the neck[65] (which is a feature of 26 per cent of all labours),[81] if the membranes are then ruptured. In these cases, the cord is then compressed between the uterine wall and the baby itself. If the cord compression lasts more than 60 seconds, the baby becomes seriously short of oxygen and will exhibit signs of distress which will require intervention.[65]

In the light of present knowledge, it would seem reasonable for mothers being admitted to hospital in labour to object to the practice of rupturing their membranes early in labour, if the only reason that can be given for it is that it may speed up the labour. The procedure is almost invariably accompanied by a change in the force and frequency of the contractions (i.e. it makes them stronger and closer together), whether or not the labour is speeded up, and it disturbs the rhythm of a labour with which the mother may be coping well until that point. Moreover, it often requires painkillers to counteract the effect of the sudden increase in intensity, which may occur in this situation long before the end of the first stage or transition. Even if rupturing the membranes in their case does cause an acceleration in labour (which is in any case a retrospective discovery), there may be a heavy price to pay in terms of iatrogenic damage. Lastly, it should be borne in mind that acceleration of labour is not necessarily beneficial for the baby. Niswander and Gordon have shown that perinatal death, and neurological damage persisting at least until the first birthday, are both increased when the duration of the first stage is shortened below a given optimal range.[82]

Monitoring

It has been known for about 150 years that the baby's heart-rate pattern changes during uterine contractions when the mother is in labour, and that while in the majority of cases these changes are a normal response of the baby to the situation, in some cases the changes may be a warning sign that all is not well with the baby. These facts form the basis for careful checking of the baby's heart rate during labour, by means of a foetal stethoscope. During the late 1960s an electronic form of foetal monitoring was introduced as an alternative to listening by ear via a stethoscope. This electronic device took two forms – external and internal – and in both cases the uterine contractions are monitored simultaneously with the baby's heart rate.

In the external version, two small devices (either flat or doughnut-shaped) are strapped to the mother's abdomen using broad rubber belts: one device is placed over the top or fundus of the uterus to record contractions, and the other over the baby's back/shoulder to record its heart rate. The two devices are connected by thin flexes to the monitor itself, which prints out the recordings of contractions and heart rate, continuously, on graph paper.

The internal version involves the attachment of a spiral needle electrode to the baby's scalp (or whichever part is over the cervix) to record the heart rate, and a plastic tube (or catheter) is inserted into the uterus, via the cervix, to record the actual pressure of the contractions via the amniotic fluid. Again, both devices are attached to the monitor by wires.

No figures are available for their relative use, but obstetric literature appears to suggest that external monitoring is less widely used because it is less reliable.[83] In some hospitals the use of electronic monitoring is backed up by foetal scalp blood sampling – that is, making a small puncture in the baby's scalp or whichever part is over the cervix – and collecting a blood sample which is then analysed to determine the oxygen concentration and the acidity or alkalinity of the blood (pH).

Once introduced, the use of electronic monitoring spread rapidly as it was claimed that it brought about considerable improvements in the infant and perinatal death rates.[84, 85] Most of these claims were based on a comparison of the mortality rates before and after the introduction of electronic foetal monitoring (EFM). Other investigations, however, showed either no difference or else a slight rise in death rates after EFM.[86] Wennberg's study in Vermont[87] showed that the decline in perinatal deaths had been the same in hospitals that had used EFM extensively as in those that had not. These studies suggest that factors other than EFM were involved in the improvement in perinatal mortality statistics. Nevertheless, a recent task force meeting at the National Institutes of Health in America estimated that 60–70 per cent of all women are monitored electronically in labour, and many obstetricians believe that this figure should be increased to 100 per cent.[83, 88]

In the midst of the debate as to the benefits of EFM, there has been a growing concern about the risks and inconveniences to the mother and baby from the use of this technique.

1.   If the mother is being monitored externally, either for contractions, foetal heart rate, or both, there is the considerable discomfort engendered by having to wear tight rubber belts throughout labour.

2.   Whether internal or external monitoring is used, unless it is being done by radiotelemetry, the mother is confined to bed and her position in bed greatly restricted by virtue of being attached by a few feet of wire, vaginally or abdominally, to the machine. This can result in decreased placental blood flow and consequent foetal distress.[89] It is also likely to make the labour longer than it need be, and to increase the mother's need for pain-relieving drugs – with subsequent repercussions for the baby (see page 101).

3.   If the mother is being monitored internally, the bag of waters surrounding the baby has to be broken to allow the introduction of a tube to record changes in pressure, and the insertion of an electrode into the baby's scalp. The consequences for both mother and baby have already been discussed (page 86), and include making the contractions sharper and closer together, increasing the degree of moulding of the baby's head, and increasing the incidence of cord and skull compression which will, in the last two cases, produce in their own right abnormal heart changes on the monitor.

4.   As might be imagined, inserting an electrode into the baby's scalp is not without its hazards. In most cases, the problems are those of scalp abscess and haemorrhage,[90-93] but there have been reports of incorrectly positioned electrodes causing lacerations to the arms, cheek, trunk and thigh,[94] due in one instance to the electrode being partially attached to the

mother's cervix; penetration of the eyelid,[95] penetration of the brain tissue causing a leak of cerebrospinal fluid,[96] and even one neonatal death, due to sepsis.[97]

5.   Less catastrophic, but very much more common, is the effect that the monitor may have on the mother's attendants: in many cases, attention that should be given to the labouring woman is given instead to the monitor, and the mother is relegated to the position of a mere generator of electrical impulses. In some instances, this is taken to the point where the monitor is given greater credibility than the mother, and if the monitor 'says' she is having weak contractions, when the mother maintains that they are strong (this may happen if the base line is incorrectly set) then the monitor is believed and the mother contradicted. This will do nothing to improve her morale, or strengthen her trust in her attendants.

6.   Whilst there are no doubt mothers who find the presence of a monitor at their bedside reassuring, there are also those who are bothered by the flashing lights, the sound produced with each heart beat and by hearing or seeing decelerations in heart rate, even when these are benign.

7.   The problem that is most consistently associated with the use of EFM is that of increased Caesarean section (with an accompanying increase in post-delivery infection).[98, 99]

In view of these possible side effects and the inadequacy of retrospective studies in deciding the possible benefits, it became apparent that the only scientific way to resolve the question of the effects of EFM was by randomized controlled clinical trials (RCTs).[100, 101] In an RCT women and their babies are randomly assigned to two different types of treatment – in this case, listening to the foetal heart via stethoscope (auscultation) or via EFM. Only four RCTs have been carried out to date: in Denver, Colorado, by Haverkamp and colleagues, from 1973–5[102] and from 1975–7;[103] in Melbourne, Australia, by Renou and colleagues in 1976;[104] and most recently in Sheffield, England, by Kelso and colleagues in 1978.[86] The first three studies all used women who were judged to be at high risk; the fourth used low-risk mothers.

None of the four studies was large enough to demonstrate any difference in perinatal mortality rates; but none of them demonstrated any differences in the Apgar scores in the two groups. The only group to publish enough information about cord blood pH to make any conclusion possible was the second Haverkamp study, which found no difference between the EFM and the auscultated group of babies. Neurological examination of the newborn babies was made in all four RCTs: the first Haverkamp study and the Kelso study found no difference at all in the two groups. The Renou study showed four babies with convulsions in the auscultated group and none in the EFM group, but it was not clear from the results whether these four were among the five who were delivered by mid-forceps, and whether therefore the convulsions should be attributed to the type of delivery, the absence of monitoring, or both. In each of these three studies, the doctors examining the babies knew to which group they belonged. The only study in which the examiners did not know in which group the babies had been was the second Haverkamp study, and this RCT reported no significant difference. This was also the only group which provided follow-up assessments at nine months of age, and again, no significant difference was found between the two groups.

Although these results are not conclusive, the RCTs appear to show no clear-cut advantage for EFM over ausculation with respect to perinatal morbidity.[105]

However, all four studies demonstrated unequivocally that there was a significant increase in the Caesarean-section rate (CSR) in the EFM group compared with the auscultated group. In the first Haverkamp study, the EFM group had a CSR of 16.5 per cent compared with 6.6 per cent for the auscultated group: in the second study, the EFM group had a CSR of 18 per cent compared with 6 per cent for the auscultated group. In the Renou study, the EFM group had a CSR of 22.3 per cent compared with 13.7 per cent, and in the Kelso study the EFM group had a CSR of 9 per cent compared with 4 per cent for the auscultated group. When all the factors except the use of EFM are controlled, there is an approximate doubling of the Caesarean-section rate as a result of using EFM.[105] This is a serious finding, for although Caesarean sections can be life-saving for mother and child, they also carry a much higher incidence of interuterine infection than vaginal deliveries, and of course also entail the increased use of anaesthesia with its own attendant risks. Two American studies have found that the risk of death from Caesarean section is 10–26 times that for vaginal delivery.[106, 107] In this country a large study has shown that in 1972 the estimated mortality from Caesarean section was more than eight times greater than from vaginal delivery.[108] As has already been shown, this increase is not offset by any improvement in perinatal mortality rate.

In their careful review of the literature (including the four RCTs quoted) Banta and Thacker concluded that there is little, if any, benefit to be derived from the use of EFM compared with auscultation. If EFM is of benefit, it appears to be confined to infants of low birth weight, but as yet there has been no RCT of EFM in this group. The risks of EFM as well as the cost to the nation are, they say, substantial. (In America the cost to society is estimated at $411 million per annum!)[105]

Because of the risks and the cost, EFM is currently being re-evaluated in America, and the newly formed National Center for Health Care will make foetal monitoring one of the first technologies which it discusses. In the meantime, in view of the problem of malpractice suits in America, the National Institute of Health task force has concluded that auscultation is an acceptable alternative to EFM in low-risk pregnancies.

If the best that can be said of electronic foetal monitoring is that it is equivalent to auscultation, perhaps we should be looking more closely at its use in this country, both in terms of unwanted side effects and in terms of the enormous cost of the machines during a period of cutback in NHS funds. Meanwhile, obstetricians must continue to make clinical decisions about their use despite the lack of evidence as to their benefits. Since some women will continue to find the presence of the monitor reassuring, while others will not, obtaining the mother's *informed* consent would appear to be the only ethical path to take.

Chapter 5

The first stage
Pain in labour

Expectation of pain in labour

Before examining in detail the drugs that are available for use
in labour, it would be logical to consider the basic assumption
made by a large proportion of the British population that
labour is necessarily and inevitably painful. When different
cultures throughout the world are compared, it is apparent
that the extent to which women expect, experience or express
(not necessarily the same thing) pain in labour varies considerably. The Navaho Indians, for example, have two distinct
words for labour. One is a word which means 'the pain of
labour', and the other 'labour' alone. There is cultural recognition of the fact that childbirth without pain is possible, and
one witness of more than 400 Navaho births has reported that
though some women definitely experienced pain, there were
also those who showed no signs of doing so.[1]

Simply comparing the drug usage rates in different populations is probably a rather crude and inaccurate measurement
of the perception of pain in labour in these populations, but
there is a dramatic difference between the United Kingdom
with a drug-usage rate in labour of 95 per cent, and Holland,
with a drug-usage rate of 5 per cent,[2] and this would suggest

that social and educational factors are also involved in the way in which labour is interpreted, and that it is not purely a matter of physiology. As Sir Henry Head, one of the great pioneer neurologists, reported in a paper published by the *British Medical Journal*, 'The mental state of the patient has a notoriously profound influence over the pain initiating in the pelvic viscera.' In other words, how the stimulus is interpreted is as relevant as the stimulus itself. Superstition, civilization and culture have all brought influences to bear upon the minds of women, and the more cultured the races of the earth have become, the more positive they have been (for the most part) in pronouncing childbirth to be a painful and dangerous ordeal. This may be due in part to the tendency in civilized societies to remove childbirth from the family setting so that it is no longer part of the flow of life, but something separate, not seen, and therefore mysterious and alarming, and also in part to the posture adopted for labour in our societies. No other animal species voluntarily assumes such disadvantageous positions during such an important and critical event as are frequently imposed upon women in Western communities.[3]

There are many fundamental ways in which a woman's expectation of the experience of labour are modified, starting from early childhood right up to the onset of labour, and it would be appropriate to look more closely at the way in which young girls – and boys – are 'taught' about labour. At the moment there seems to be comparatively little available to counteract the disastrous effects of descriptions of childbirth in many works of fiction, and worse still, television, films and plays, where birth is represented (as opposed to recorded); these last three are much more effortlessly and insidiously absorbed. If a child watches a programme in which a woman supposedly giving birth lies flat, in a bed, hanging on to the sides or the headrails, rigid and screaming, and the attendants act as though this is appropriate behaviour, it is likely that this will leave a lasting impression on the child's mind. If this is not balanced out by good, factual information from parents or schools or, worse still, if the effects are compounded by half-heard conversations about a neighbour's or relative's 'awful time', then it is not surprising that the adult the child grows into views childbirth with extreme trepidation.

The situation may be improved by good antenatal preparation, including information, relaxation and breathing techniques appropriate for dealing with the stresses of labour, received by the now more mature mind of the expectant parent, but even so the antenatal teacher cannot hope to correct in eight to ten weeks the impressions and misconceptions which have been accumulated over the years. 'What . . . [women] . . . bring to labour is nothing less than [their] entire socialization as women.'[4] It is worth looking closely at the physiological and psychological factors that influence the subjective experience of labour.

There are three layers of muscle fibres in the wall of the uterus which, while not anatomically separate, have different functions. The longitudinal fibres run from the cervix, or neck of the uterus, up to the top (fundus) of the uterus and down the other side. When these contract, they shorten the uterus, and are therefore mainly used in the expulsive, second stage. The spiral or oblique fibres also start at the cervix and run in all directions in the body of the uterus so that when these contract during labour they play a major part in 'taking up' or shortening the elongated cervix and then dilating it until it is eventually wide enough to allow the baby's head to pass down into the vagina without obstruction – when it is said to be fully dilated. During and after the separation of the placenta (afterbirth) these fibres, by virtue of being entwined in a figure-of-eight fashion around the larger blood vessels, help to reduce the blood loss after the baby is born. The circular fibres, as the name implies, pass in a horizontal manner round the uterus, mainly in the lower half of the uterus and the cervix. When these contract, they tend to close the cervix and inhibit the activity of the lower part of the uterus during labour.

The precise nerve supply to the uterus is incompletely understood but the uterus seems to be supplied principally by autonomic nerves from the lumbar and pelvic ganglia, but it may be also that the logitudinal and oblique fibres are supplied by local ganglia within the uterus, unconnected with the spinal cord or autonomic system. Certainly the uterus can continue to contract when the autonomic system is cut off.[5] In practice, in a smoothly coordinated labour, the longitudinal and spiral muscles contract and start to open the cervix, and the circular fibres around the cervix stay relaxed to allow this to happen. Simple, unopposed muscle contraction does not in itself produce pain. The only pain receptors in the abdomen are those which detect excessive tension in, or tearing of, the tissues. The intestines and uterus can be burnt (cauterized), handled or moved without any sensation of pain, but if either of these structures is stretched or torn considerable pain and shock may result. The pain perceived in labour therefore must result from one or both of these specific stimuli.

If a woman has been led to expect pain, then she is likely to be in a state of tension, 'waiting for the pain'. This diffuse state will increase the intensity of the (new) sensations of labour and thus tend to bring her defence (fight-or-flight) mechanisms into operation. The same chain reaction occurs if she is frightened, or alarmed, whether by internal or external events. This release of adrenaline has the same effect as the stimulation of the sympathetic nervous system and two things happen. First, the circular fibres of the uterus start to contract in direct opposition to the contracting oblique and longitudinal fibres, and a tug-of-war begins. This rapidly produces a state of abnormal tension in the walls of the uterus which is in turn recorded by the receptors specific for that form of stimulation, and is correctly interpreted as pain. Now she has involuntarily justified her original apprehension and the vicious circle of fear–tension–pain as described by Grantly Dick Read is set up.[6]

The other effect of sympathetic stimulation is to reduce the blood flow to organs not needed for defence, and divert it to the heart, lungs and skeletal muscles. Thus the uterus, not being required for defence, subsequently has its blood supply reduced, in spite of the fact that it is actively contracting. The fact that restricting the circulation to an actively contracting muscle produces pain is well known (e.g. in angina) and can be simply demonstrated by rapidly opening and closing the fist of one hand whilst restricting the blood supply at the wrist with the other. The explanation for the pain in physiological terms was put forward by Sir Thomas Lewis,[7] who suggested that in such circumstances the breakdown products of tissue respiration accumulate faster than the blood stream can remove them, so that they build up in crystalline form, lacerating the walls of the blood sinuses and smaller vessels within the muscle fibres. If a restricted blood supply is allowed to persist for any length of time, the baby within the uterus is also likely to be deprived of oxygen, producing foetal distress, possibly brain damage, and even intrauterine death.

The powerful effect of fear and tension on the physiological process of parturition is well illustrated in the animal kingdom. The labouring female red deer, if frightened during labour, can actually cause her contractions to slow down and stop, by creating so much tension in her muscles and glands that they cease to function. She can now move away from the source of potential danger, and once she has found another quiet spot and allows her body to relax, her contractions begin again unhindered (Professor C. Naaktgeboren). Other animals are not quite so good at successfully stopping the process and starting it again without ill effects. In sheep, for instance, any unnatural disturbance during labour produces a considerable increase in the number of deliveries in which the assistance of the veterinary surgeon is required, and in cattle, dogs and rats not only do such disturbances prolong labour, but also result in a much higher perinatal mortality rate.[8]

A frequent observed phenomenon in hospitals is that of the woman who starts experiencing regular contractions at home and is admitted to hospital in labour, only to discover that her contractions have stopped. Even if the woman has no conscious fear of hospitals and believes that it is necessary for her to give birth in one, the changing surroundings appear to exert a powerful influence on her inner biological rhythm. It may be relevant here also to quote Grantly Dick Read's comments on the prolonged labour syndrome – speaking of course of those cases where there is no disproportion or malpresentation of the baby. He says that 'A labour . . . is long because it is painful, not painful because it is long.'[6]

Many factors may trigger this unhappy state of affairs, both in pregnancy and in labour. Antenatal classes which teach relaxation but stress the availability of drugs for 'when it gets too bad' or for 'when the breathing isn't enough' reinforce the inevitability of pain. The suggestion of pain is conveyed by the atmosphere of many labour and delivery rooms, which look like operating theatres: it emanates from doctors, midwives, nurses and relatives. If they all believe in pain, then subconsciously or consciously they suggest, expect and even presume pain. Upon the sensitive mind of the woman in labour, looks of sympathy, exhortations to 'be brave', or even 'not to be a martyr' are all powerful pain producers.

Dr Peter Dunn has remarked in a paper published in the *Lancet* that, 'It is my belief that the misunderstanding of this subject [pain in labour] and the use of analgesics as the first line of defence is one of the saddest developments in obstetrics.'[3]

Most of the world's mothers receive few or no drugs in labour or delivery. The constant emotional support provided by familiar people, friends, relatives or midwives is the commonest cross-cultural resource for dealing with the powerful experience of labour, and appears to improve considerably the mother's tolerance to discomfort and raise her pain threshold. In such societies the labouring woman has a greater confidence in her own ability to give birth unaided than is usually the case in ours: her attendants keep her morale high and bring no fear to the normal process. In contrast, the labour room nurse/midwife in Britain and America is frequently assigned to look after several women in labour and in this situation, particularly if the labouring woman has received no preparation in coping with the sensations of labour, drugs are used as a substitute for emotional support, to relieve the mother's apprehension, discomfort and eventually pain, and perhaps to assuage the harried labour attendant's feelings of inadequacy.[9]

It is an indictment of modern obstetric practice that it is possible to look through the case notes for a record of drugs administered in labour and to observe, not what sort of pain the woman had, but which consultant she was under or which midwife was on duty.[2, 10]

Sedating a woman not only makes her quieter and easier to manage, and gives the midwife or doctor the feeling that they have done something to 'improve' the situation, it also subdues the feelings of helplessness and anxiety generated in themselves by the woman's response to her labour. If the labour attendant is unable to offer emotional support through personal inadequacy, lack of training or lack of time, and the woman is also deprived of those who can offer them – husbands, friends and other labour companions – then analgesics will appear superficially to provide the same effect.

On the other hand, there are those who see no point at all in withholding drugs if they are available, and are unable to entertain the idea that a labour might simply involve hard work rather than pain. 'Why should she be allowed to continue to suffer?' they ask themselves, observing a woman in labour, and in many cases totally fail to interpret correctly the signals given out by the woman concentrating hard on the sensations of the late first stage, which are saying, 'Support me – tell me this is supposed to happen,' and not, as they mistakenly read them, 'Stop all this – do it for me.'[11]

Part of this attitude may be explained by the training received by midwives. In the 1950s, the teaching was that at a particular stage of labour, a certain quantity of a certain drug was given as routine, and the idea that some women might not require analgesia was never entertained. Even now, very little is included in the training given to midwives on the alternatives to drugs.

The purpose of this chapter has been to underline the premise that pain is neither necessary nor inevitable in a normal labour. However, whilst it may be possible to prevent a woman from perceiving her labour as painful by the understanding and implementation of the principles discussed, it is quite another matter to reverse the situation, non-pharmaco-

logically, when pain exists: when there are underlying physiological causes such as disproportion, malpresentation, it may
be impossible. It would in any case be cruel to deny the
validity of the woman's subjective experience of pain (even in
normal labour) on the grounds that it was physiologically
'unnecessary'. It may well be 'all in the mind', but it is none
the less real. This being so, the next consideration is of the
drugs currently used in obstetrics, the argument here being
that the potential recipient should be fully aware of the hazards of any drugs, as well as the benefits, that they should
be used highly selectively, and with her full knowledge and
consent.[2]

Pharmacological methods of pain relief in labour

In a few instances the use of pain-relieving drugs in labour is
indicated on medical grounds, such as epidural anaesthesia
where the mother's blood pressure is very high, or, more
rarely, when her response to pain threatens the welfare of
herself and her baby, e.g. overbreathing (hyperventilation).
In this instance, if a mother breathes too rapidly and deeply
as a result of the pain she is experiencing, she breathes out
more carbon dioxide (waste gas) than her body needs to get
rid of, and she starts to feel faint, then gets a tingling sensation
in her fingers and feet, which may eventually start to curl up
involuntarily and go into spasm. As a result, the oxygen
supply to the baby may be reduced and, if the mother cannot
correct this herself by breathing in and out of cupped hands
or a paper bag, then it would be appropriate to institute
pharmacological methods of pain relief as a matter of urgency.

In most cases, drugs are offered to a labouring woman to
relieve the pain or discomfor that her attendants *assume* she
is experiencing. Even if they are correct in their assumption,
it is vital that the mother's wishes are respected and her
consent obtained. 'Informed consent sometimes has the effect
of alarming a patient, and then taking up the doctor's/mid-
wife's time while her fears are put into perspective – but
anything less is not informed consent, it is selling.'[12] On her

individual refusal or acceptance of drugs offered may depend the quality of her labour (and her memory of it), the quality and type of her delivery, and more extremely, the condition of her baby and the quality of its future life. It is important that a mother is aware of her right to refuse drugs when they are suggested solely for her comfort, and that this is not an area where anyone else can possibly know better what would be 'good' for her, since only she knows what she is feeling. The other very important consideration is the possible side effects that the proposed drug may have. It is astonishing that so much publicity is given to the dangers of smoking and drug-taking in pregnancy, and so little to the possible dangers of using narcotics and other drugs in labour. Being in labour confers no sudden barrier-like properties on the placenta, and virtually all drugs given in labour tend to cross the placenta rapidly and alter the foetal environment as they enter the circulatory system of the unborn infant, within minutes or seconds of being administered to the mother.[13] Even if this had not been shown, it would seem logical to assume that any drug which could affect the mother's central nervous system would also cross the placenta and affect the baby's nervous system. The added problem with drug administration in labour is the fact that although whilst the baby is in utero the mother's liver is still involved in detoxifying any circulating drugs, if the baby is *born* with any of the drugs in his bloodstream, he is then dependent on his own liver to complete the process of detoxification. As is well known, the neonate's liver is one of the last systems to mature, so that timing of a drug is as important as the type and dose; a drug like pethidine, for instance, which the mother can clear in a matter of hours may persist in the baby for several days. At best, the drugs given to the mother will have a minimal or negligible effect on her baby; certainly they will have no beneficial effect.[14]

As far as the mother herself is concerned, it would be wrong for her to assume, or for her attendants to assure her, that drugs administered by a midwife or doctor are in any way guaranteed to have the effect that is intended, or that there are no risks involved. In order for her to be able to make a decision about the use of any particular drug in labour, she needs to know as much as possible *antenatally* about the benefits and hazards of the range available both for her and for her baby.

If a mother decided that in her particular circumstances in labour the advantages of accepting a particular drug despite its possible side effects still outweigh the disadvantages of doing without it, then that is her choice and one that she is perfectly entitled to make. Moreover, the much repeated exhortation not to 'feel a failure' if drugs are used is unlikely to be relevant, since the mother will be able to justify her decision to herself.

The problems arise when the mother who is ignorant of the possible hazards accepts a particular drug and then discovers later the implications of having done so. It is necessary to keep in mind that it is the mother who must ultimately bear the emotional burden of the decision, particularly if the child is damaged or impaired. 'As the public becomes more aware of the possible effects of obstetric practices on infant outcome, failure to disclose or inform the mother of the possible adverse consequences . . . may become the basis of legal liability if or when those adverse consequences occur.'[15]

The following is an examination of the drugs commonly used in labour. (It cannot be overstressed that vaginal examination to assess the dilation of the cervix should *precede* the administration of any drug or other form of intervention.)

Pethidine

This is a synthetic narcotic introduced in 1940 as an alternative to heroin and morphine. It is known as meperidine or Demerol in the USA. Its popularity evolved from the mistaken belief that pethidine was an 'antispasmodic' which would both relieve pain and relax the uterus, the latter in contrast to morphine.[16] It can be given in quantities of 50 mg, 100 mg, 150 mg, or 200 mg at a time, and although the initial authorization has to be made by a doctor, this may be done in the case of midwives working in a GP unit weeks in advance of labour, and is administered largely at the discretion of the midwife. Domiciliary midwives are empowered by the CMB to administer pethidine on their own authority. It is given by intramuscular injection.

Maternal advantages   Pethidine is given with the intention of helping the labouring woman to relax more easily, and by inducing a sensation of distance or separation from reality, helping her to cope better with the contractions. It is not intended to remove pain altogether. It is sometimes used in the belief that it will lower blood pressure.

Maternal disadvantages   If the above effect is taken a little further, it may make the mother too drowsy to register anything more than the peak of the contractions, making her unable to prepare for them, and thus removing what little control she has over her labour. Taken further still, it may make the mother go to sleep, waking only when the drug starts to wear off. It has no direct effect on uterine action, but it has been observed to slow down labour in some cases.[17] In 15 per cent of cases it induces nausea or vomiting, and is thus frequently combined with an anti-emetic (see below). It is not a good analgesic, and in a double-blind trial quoted by Martin Richards[18] only 52 per cent of women could distinguish between pethidine and saline administered intramuscularly. In another trial,[19] only 50–60 per cent of mothers regarded the analgesic effect to be satisfactory. If the mother is to be made drowsy without obtaining any analgesic benefit, then the situation is made worse than before as far as she is concerned, even though it may make her 'easier' for her attendants to manage. Unfortunately, too, it is not possible to predict in advance the effect of pethidine on a particular mother: 50 mg may send one mother to sleep, and have no effect at all on another. For this reason it would be advisable for any mother not familiar with the effects of pethidine in herself to request that she be given only 50 mg to start with (despite the belief that a dose of less than 50 mg is indistinguishable from a placebo)[20], on the grounds that she can always have some more later if 50 mg proves to be ineffective.

(Some midwives in America start with doses as low as 25 mg, and never expect to use more than 75 mg.) There is nothing she can do to rid herself of the excess drug if she is given too much for her needs, except to wait until it wears off – in one and a half to two hours.

Disadvantages to the baby   It has now been well established that pethidine, in common with pethilorphan, barbiturates, some tranquillizers and epidurals, has an effect on the baby's ability to suck[21] which is not necessarily related to its Apgar score (see pages 67–8). In extreme cases this may actually inhibit lactation.[22] It may also make the baby dopy, sleepy and slow to breathe, and the effects on sucking may last for up to two weeks.[18]

It is also well established that pethidine has an effect on the baby's ability to habituate, that is, to acclimatize itself to a particular repeated stimulus and then ignore it if it is not relevant. A newborn baby whose mother has received no drugs in labour may take five to six exposures to the same stimulus – i.e. a noise or a shining light – before he ignores it. A baby whose mother has received pethidine may need 13 to 15 exposures to the same stimulus before he can ignore it. Pethidine delays the development of the ability to habituate for at least two months[18] and the overall effect of pethidine on the newborn may be the unfortunately familiar sight in some maternity hospitals of the baby who is at the same time jumpy and sleepy, and a poor feeder in addition! Such babies are difficult to handle and may undermine the confidence of the mother, especially if it is her first baby, with subsequent deleterious effects on the mother–infant relationship if she feels that she can do nothing right. Brackbill, in her study of mother–infant interaction, states that 'meperidine (pethidine) produces outstanding neonatal differences in the ability to process information' and that to her 'a major obstetric danger may now be medication itself.'[23, 24]

Apart from the dose, and the maturity of the infant (and narcotics especially should be avoided in preterm deliveries), the effects of pethidine will also depend on the timing. It is widely held that the dose should be administered four hours before the birth to have the minimal effect on the baby. However, measurements of the excretion of pethidine in the baby's urine indicate that the concentration continues to increase for up to five hours,[25] and it also appears that the side effects are produced not just by the pethidine itself but by a breakdown product of pethidine also, so that the drug would need to be given six to eight hours before delivery to have the minimal effect – or one to two hours before delivery, in which case the mother might well go to sleep immediately after the birth. In the former case, six to eight hours would be somewhat difficult to estimate. Four hours before delivery, however, is probably the worst possible time for administration.[18, 26]

Pethilorphan

This is a mixture of pethidine and a narcotic anatagonist, levallorphan. This drug is also given by intramuscular injection and was used in 25 per cent of labours in 1970[27] – this despite the publication of a number of studies showing that for the mother it is less effective than pethidine as an analgesic[28] and had pethidine's disadvantages.

Disadvantages to the baby   These are similar to those of pethidine, except that the inclusion of levallorphan, which has been shown to have a much more depressive effect,[29] makes them worse: the babies suffer from mild respiratory depression and are slower to cry and breathe at birth.[30] Abnormal neurobehavioural effects, such as habituation retardation, have been reported at much later intervals than with pethidine.[31] At 30 weeks and again at 60 weeks babies and mothers have less intimate contact with each other and babies show more self-stimulatory activities such as thumb-sucking. Martin Richards comments that 'It is unlikely that an event that has led to a different path of development in the first 12 months will not continue to have some influence.'[30]

Tranquillizers

These are given to allay anxiety and reduce tension. The two most commonly used are Valium (diazepam) and Sparine (promazine). Valium is widely used as a tranquillizer and in the treatment of pre-eclampsia in pregnancy in an attempt to lower blood pressure. Sparine is used for the same reason in labour, to reduce blood pressure by reducing anxiety, and also helps to reduce the nauseant side effects of pethidine. Tranquillizers in general, and Valium in particular, have a direct effect on muscle tone in the newborn (hypotonia) and reduce the ability to breathe at birth and the ability to suck; they may also have the effect of profoundly reducing body temperature (hypothermia).[32] Both these effects may last for days or weeks and in the view of many paediatricians these drugs have little place in obstetrics.[18]

Phenothiazine derivatives

Fentazin (perphenazine) and Phenergan (promethazine) are usually used in labour to counteract the nauseant side effects of pethidine. They both have a sedative side effect and react with pethidine, so that the sum total of their effect is greater than that of simple addition (synergism),[32] Phenergan also having been shown in one study to disturb the ability of the baby's blood to clot.[33]

Inhalation analgesia ('gas and air')

The two most commonly used inhalation analgesics are 0.35 per cent methoxyfluorane in air (Penthrane) and 50 per cent nitrous oxide with 50 per cent oxygen (Entonox) of which the latter seems to be the more popular. Both are potentially general anaesthetics, but are administered in subanaesthetic concentrations through systems that make self-administration possible. If the mother takes too much and falls asleep, then the mask slips down from her face: she breathes air and wakes up (one very good reason why the mask should never be forcibly held over the mother's face, unfortunately not an uncommon sight in some institutions). In both cases the successful use depends on the mother's learning how to make the peak concentration of the agent in her blood coincide with the peak of a contraction, and this is best done by antenatal instruction and experimentation under supervision.

The advantages to the mother are that the effects are immediate and short-lived. If she finds it useful, and the majority of those who use it (70 per cent for Entonox[34] and 90 per cent for Penthrane[35]) find it *is* useful, she can continue to self-administer it, and if she dislikes its effect she can discontinue it and the effects will have worn off within a minute. These two inhalation analgesics may also be useful in reducing the effects of overbreathing. Penthrane, being a soluble agent, stays in the blood longer, thus making it easier to ensure successful peak pain relief, but that is also its disadvantage, as over 30 per cent of it is metabolized and the breakdown product, a fluoride compound, may damage the kidneys if present in large amounts, though this is unlikely with the low concentration level used. Entonox, being insoluble, is almost totally excreted via the lungs during contractions, but this means it is more difficult to get the timing right. The fact that the mother can, in both cases control the gas and air machine herself is, however, of great psychological advantage.

There have been no studies done on the effects of inhalation analgesia alone on the infant, since it is so often used in conjunction with pethidine. Penthrane usage, however, has been shown to result in an increased fluoride concentration in the baby's urine for up to 48 hours.[36] Entonox appears to have no measurable effect on the baby.[18] There appear to be no indications to limit the duration of administration and theoretically Entonox at least could be used throughout labour and is a much undervalued analgesic.

Local anaesthetic agents used in labour

Pudendal nerve block   The pudendal nerves supply most of the perineum, vulva, vagina and muscles of the pelvic floor. The nerves in the side walls of the pelvis are injected with local anaesthetic thus numbing the area completely. It is easy to perform and usually successful, and is done to provide local anaesthesia prior to an instrumental vaginal delivery. The disadvantages to both mother and child are that large quantities are required to produce the necessary effect, and this can result in overdose.[37]

Paracervical block   This is an injection of local anaesthetic into the pelvic uterine plexuses which supply the nerves to most of the cervix and uterus. The advantages to the mother are that this technique provides satisfactory analgesia for (and shortens) the first stage of labour for the majority of women, but the disadvantages are so great for the baby that, despite its continued use in some centres, particularly in Scandinavia and America, Rosen regards it as 'not now recommended'.[37] Several studies[38] have reported severe changes in heart rate, respiration and muscle tone in over 30 per cent of babies where their mothers had this technique used. According to one study presented at the International Symposium on the Effect of Prolonged Drug Usage on Foetal Development, 1971, 'Foetal depression, even if apparently reversible, might later affect the motor and intellectual development of the child.' The fact that babies actually do die as a result of paracervical blocks has also been clearly demonstrated.[39]

Lumbar epidural anaesthesia   This is an injection of local anaesthetic into the epidural or extradural space. (This space is outside the last of the three membranes which cover the spinal cord, and just inside the bone and ligament of the vertebral column.) It must not be adminstered except by a skilled practitioner, who should remain on the premises in case complications such as spinal block should occur. The process, which is a sterile procedure, takes 10–20 minutes to complete, and begins with the setting up of an intravenous infusion (drip) of dextrose (sugar) in water. This is in case the fall in blood pressure caused inevitably by the epidural needs to be reversed rapidly by intravenous means. The mother is then asked to lie on her left side, in as much of a ball as possible, with her back as close as possible to the edge of the bed. She is asked to inform the anaesthetist when she is experiencing a contraction, so that he may temporarily halt the procedure, and she may be given gas and air to breathe. She will then feel the pressure of the anaesthetist's thumbs on her back as he feels for the necessary bony landmarks. Her back is washed with a very cold spirit solution, and then a very small central skin area in the lumbar region is injected with local anaesthetic which stings for a few seconds and then produces a feeling of numbness. All the mother should be aware of now is a pushing sensation against her back, until the process is nearly complete. What the anaesthetist is doing is firstly making a small hole through the skin and ligaments with a solid needle. This is then removed, and a hollow needle with a syringe half full of air is inserted in its place. The hollow needle is pushed in slowly until the plunger on the syringe gives, indicating that there is no longer any resistance at the point of the needle. The syringe is then taken off and the end of the hollow needle is observed for a few seconds: if the needle has been pushed in too far and the dura punctured, this should be apparent at this stage, as spinal fluid would drip out of the needle (accidental lumbar puncture). Assuming all is well, a fine, soft catheter is then threaded down through the needle. This may cause a slight twinge down one leg momentarily. When the catheter has been threaded far enough, the hollow needle is removed, leaving just a long length of catheter protruding from the skin. The point of entry is then sealed, using plastic skin, a small sponge pad placed around this and the external part of the catheter is secured to the skin along the whole of its length, using paper tape (to prevent sticking plaster reaction). This is continued up the back to the shoulder, or sometimes up to the abdomen. A small filter and a 'bung' are then attached to the end of the catheter and a test dose of local anaesthetic can then be given by syringe down the catheter via the filter, followed by a full dose, and the uterus and cervix anaesthetized. If high concentrations of local anaesthetic are used, there may be some loss of muscle power also. This effect usually lasts for one and a half to two hours, but can be 'topped up' as often as necessary throughout labour. The epidural catheter can be inserted before the onset of labour, in the case of induction if required, with no limitation of the mother's movement, but once the anaesthetic agent has been given, the mother is instructed to lie on her side, because of the potential effect on her blood pressure, which is checked very frequently thereafter.

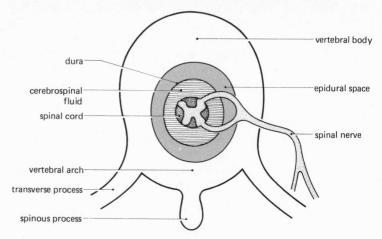

transverse section of spinal column

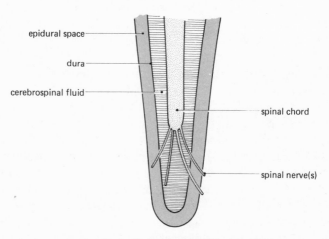

longitudinal section of spinal column

Maternal advantages

1. When properly effective, lumbar epidural anaesthesia provides complete pain relief without dulling the mother's mental faculties.

2. It may be of benefit to mothers with serious heart or respiratory disease, as it reduces the work of the lungs in labour.

3. As it reduces muscle activity, it may be of value in the case of a diabetic mother, by reducing her metabolic demands and making it easier to balance her insulin and glucose requirements.

4. As it has the tendency to slow down labour,[40] it may be of value in the management of very rapid (precipitate) labour.

5. Where problems may arise with a very premature pushing urge, e.g. footling breech, an epidural may be helpful.

6. As an alternative to a pudendal block, where forceps or vacuum extraction is necessary.

7. It often provides an effective means of lowering the blood pressure where pre-eclamptic toxaemia or hypertension is a problem.

8. In some centres elective Caesarean sections can be performed using epidural instead of general anaesthesia. This means that the mother can be conscious for the operation and can see and hold her baby immediately after its birth.

Maternal disadvantages

1. The epidurals may be ineffective or only partially effective in removing the sensation of the contractions. This is a serious psychological complication because if the mother is promised that it will 'all be over' for her in terms of coping with the contractions in 10 to 15 minutes, she will mentally give up her grip on her labour and her responsibility for coping with it. If the promised relief does not then materialize, she is in

the distressing position of having mentally to take the reins again, which may have a devastating effect on her morale.

2. Accidental lumbar puncture. This occurs on average in 1–2 per cent of epidural administration.[41] Because of the size of the hollow needle, quite a large hole may be made in the dura if the needle is pushed too far. This may result in severe headache which will require the mother to lie flat in bed for at least forty-eight hours after delivery, and treatment entails the infusion of fluid into the epidural space to raise the pressure and close the hole. Sometimes 5–10 ml of the mother's own blood is injected into the epidural space to stop the leak of spinal fluid. Pain relief may be obtained by giving analgesics (which may have their own complications if the mother is breast-feeding) or by inhaling 5 per cent carbon dioxide with 95 per cent oxygen for four to five minutes, although this provides only temporary relief.

3. Accidental subarachnoid injection. This occurs if the catheter itself punctures the dura when it is being threaded down the hollow needle. It may not be immediately obvious when the test dose is given, but the effect of giving the full dose (five or more times that intended for spinal anaesthesia – see page 116) is that of a widespread block which may involve the muscles of respiration, paralysing them so that emergency artificial ventilation becomes necessary.

4. Postdelivery neurological complications. These are fairly unusual, but mothers do occasionally complain of numbness in the legs or weakness and difficulty in walking or cycling. These symptoms do not last more than a few weeks, but may obviously cause the mother considerable concern. The only cases of permanent paralysis as a result of faulty technique that have been recorded were twenty years ago, as a result of infection prior to the use of adequate aseptic procedures.[41]

5. Hypotension (lowering of the blood pressure). Although this is one of the advantages of an epidural when the blood pressure is abnormally high, it becomes a disadvantage when the labouring woman has normal or low blood pressure. As

well as blocking a section of spinal nerves, an effective epidural also blocks off a section of autonomic ganglia which control the ability of blood vessels supplied by them to constrict, thus raising the blood pressure. When a woman lies flat on her back in late pregnancy or labour, the weight of her pregnant uterus compresses a major blood vessel returning blood to the heart, which would potentially lead to a lowering of the volume of blood pumped out by the heart and a fall in blood pressure. In 85 per cent of the pregnant population the compensatory constriction of the blood vessels keeps the blood pressure normal. The other 15 per cent are unable to compensate effectively and their blood pressure drops (supine hypotension). By giving the labouring woman an epidural, the anaesthetist is depriving her of the ability to counteract the effects of a drop in blood pressure, should it occur, and for this reason no woman with an epidural should ever be allowed to lie flat unsupervised. Maternal deaths have been recorded when this precaution has been overlooked.[41] Sometimes the blood pressure falls dangerously even when the mother is not lying flat, and large quantities of fluid have to be given intravenously, via the intravenous infusion system which should already be in progress.

6. Forceps delivery. A fully effective epidural in the second stage greatly increases the incidence of forceps delivery. The woman cannot feel when her uterus is pushing, and if she is *told* by her attendants and goes through the motions of pushing, she has no feedback from her vagina and perineum to guide her. In addition, there may be a loss of muscle power, depending on the concentration of anaesthetic agent used. She is likely to make much slower progress in the second stage in this situation, and if there is an arbitrary limit on the second stage, irrespective of the condition of mother and baby, then the incidence of forceps delivery will be higher still. The incidence of forceps delivery among women having first babies was shown in the 1977 Oxford Epidural Study[42] to be 70 per cent, and for second and subsequent babies 40 per cent. The time of administration (i.e. early or late in labour) made no

difference. If the epidural were allowed to wear off as the second stage progressed, and the mother could feel what she was doing, then the forceps rate dropped considerably, but it was still higher than if she had not had an epidural (20 per cent). The reason for this is the decrease in tone of the muscles of the pelvic floor. In their normal, unrelaxed state they form a gutter shape which serves to guide the baby's head as it descends and causes it to rotate towards the front. This mechanism is interfered with when an epidural is given, and cannot be reversed by allowing the epidural to wear off. The authors[42] suggest that further study is needed into the possible trauma that might occur to both mother and child if 20 per cent of all mothers having epidural anaesthesia have to be delivered by Kiellands (rotation) forceps.

In some units all babies delivered by forceps, for whatever reason, spend a period in the intensive care nursery, which results in early separation of mother and child. It has been suggested that [42] in the absence of strong medical indications for regional anaesthesia, the mother should be made aware of the increased chance of instrumental delivery, so that she could herself choose between such a method of pain relief and the considerably reduced chance of a spontaneous delivery.

7. Bladder complications. No complications arise as a result of the epidural itself, but the resultant loss of normal sensation following epidural may necessitate catheterization, that is the passage of a soft polythene or rubber tube up the urethra and into the bladder to drain the urine during labour; the more often this is done, the greater is the likelihood of bladder infection and irritation of the urethra, resulting in increased difficulty for the mother in passing urine after delivery. In some cases this may necessitate a rubber catheter being left in for one to two days while the swelling and irritation subside.

Contraindications

The following contraindications to an epidural block should also be considered:

1. The mother may not want the procedure.

2. There may be an area of infection near the proposed site.

3. The mother may be taking anticoagulants, or have a bleeding disorder.

4. She may have had a substantial bleed from the uterus prior to labour (antepartum haemorrhage) or be likely to bleed.

5. The mother may have neurological or spine disease or injury.

6. It has been suggested by McDonald *et al.* that the use of epidural anaesthesia should be restricted where there is a reason to suspect 'foetal compromise' as in severe pre-eclampsia or postmaturity when associated with placental insufficiency, as they found that even small doses (given to mothers in whom low blood pressure was not a problem) produced changes in foetal heart pattern (due to the depressant effect of the local anaesthetic on heart muscle) that corresponded with those found in foetal hypoxia (oxygen shortage).[43]

Disadvantages to the baby

1. If the mother's blood pressure is allowed to drop as a result of epidural administration, and the amount of blood and therefore oxygen supplying the placenta is reduced, foetal bradycardia (a slowing down of the baby's heart rate) may occur, particularly if the mother is lying flat, and this is made worse if oxytocin is being used.[44] How much the baby's oxygen supply can be reduced before neurological damage ensues may not be recognized for many years.

2. Since there are blood vessels in the epidural space, the local anaesthetic present can be absorbed into the mother's blood stream and thus transferred to the baby via the placenta. The degree to which this happens depends on the type and quantity of the local anaesthetic used. Some types cause slowing of the baby's heart rate,[45] a reduction in the oxygen available to the baby and an increase in the acidity of its blood.[26, 46] Others produce poor muscle tone, which has been shown to affect the baby's ability to suck, unrelated to its Apgar score.[18, 41, 47]

3. If the baby has to be delivered by forceps or vacuum extraction purely as a result of the type of analgesia used for the mother, and not for any underlying mechanical difficulties, then this can reasonably be regarded as a disadvantage.

Spinal anaesthesia

This is a small quantity of local anaesthetic injected into the tissue space immediately surrounding the spinal cord. It is usually given only once, and is used mainly as an alternative to pudendal blocks and epidurals to provide anaesthesia for forceps or vacuum extraction deliveries. It has the advantage of needing only a small quantity of local anaesthetic, so that the possibility of overdose for the mother or toxicity for the baby are reduced. However, it has the disadvantages of causing a possible drop in blood pressure and severe headaches after delivery (see page 112) as the needle must pass through the dura. It is not very widely used in Britain.

Chapter 6

The second stage

The requirement for the woman to assume the lithotomy position for delivery

The lithotomy position is one in which the woman lies flat on her back on the bed/delivery table with her knees drawn up and spread apart, often with her feet in stirrups.

Since it was first advocated in print in 1824 by Dewees,[1] considerable research has been done on the problems it engenders. The recumbent position, as has already been mentioned (see page 48) was advocated to facilitate the use of forceps and to give the accoucheur ready access to the perineum. The arguments used in that section to demonstrate the ill effects which follow if the labouring woman lies flat on her back in the first stage of labour are equally applicable in the second – namely, the lowering of maternal blood pressure, the reduction in the volume of blood flowing back to the heart, and the potential drop in oxygen supply to the baby.

The aorta, inferior vena cava, iliac arteries and ureters are all capable of being compressed between the spine and the uterus, causing complete disturbance of the mother's circulation and urine output, which in turn have an unfavourable and distressing effect on the foetus.[2]

Among the other ill effects which follow from the assumption of the lithotomy position are greater pain in the second stage of labour, greater incidence of perineal tears and/or episi-otomy, increased need for forceps, increased traction when forceps are used, inhibition of spontaneous placental delivery, and greater likelihood of low back strain following delivery.

Greater pain

Lusk, writing in 1894, stated that 'During the second stage the patient's posture should be left in general to her own volition.' From the subjective point of view, the best position is likely to be that which results in the minimum of pain and discomfort for the mother. It is also likely to be the most advantageous for delivery from the mechanical point of view.[3] Howard[4] who in 1954 designed a back rest for the delivery table so that mothers could sit up, claimed that, 'Even now, the majority of humans are born physiologically and for the most part in the squatting position or a variation thereof.' He regarded the supine or lithotomy position in general use by modern Western physicians as abnormal and 'unphysiologic'. This prompted an investigation of the Human Relations Area Files by Naroll *et al.* in 1961.[5] (These files are a collection of hundreds of first-hand reports about a large sample of human societies from all over the world: the files are so arranged that the original text of any passage which deals with childbirth in any of the reports can be quickly located and consulted.[6,7])

They defined 'upright' as a position in which 'a line con-necting the centres of a woman's third and fifth lumbar ver-tebrae was more nearly horizontal than vertical' and in such a way that the third vertebra was higher than the fifth.

Whilst noting that 'primitive peoples display a wider variety of culture patterns than civilized peoples', so that no one position could be singled out as 'normal', they found that 62 out of the 76 non-Western cultures they studied used an upright position; 21, some kind of kneeling position; 15, some kind of squatting position; 5 stood, and 19 used a sitting position. Since these peoples are not constrained by Western obstetrics, it is reasonable to assume that they adopt these positions because they want to do so – because it is more comfortable. This contention is further supported by a personal communication from Newton (Professor of Obstetrics at the University of Mississippi) to Howard[4] in which Newton stated that he was looking for a way to achieve more comfort in delivery in a group of underprivileged women who could not afford the expense of analgesia or anaesthesia. This was accomplished by allowing them to assume an upright position.[8] In a later study by Newton, covering 349 mothers, he found that those who were upright required less analgesia for delivery than the controls (132) who were lying down – this irrespective of the number of children they had already borne.[9]

The increased need for forceps

This is likely to be due in part to the greater need for analgesia if the woman is flat, see above, (epidural anaesthesia in particular has been shown to result in a dramatic increase in the forceps rate),[10] and in part due to the effect of the supine position on the mechanics of the second stage.

Professor Mendez-Bauer[11] estimated that the force of gravity in the upright position was equivalent alone to a continuous uterine contractile force of 30–40 mmHg – and that this increased efficiency was achieved without any increase in the incidence of foetal distress.[12] If the mother is lying flat, she is pushing her baby out at right angles to the gravitational force. This results in a greater incidence of tearing (see pages 141–2) as the resultant force is directed at the perineum rather than the vagina, but also results in considerably more effort on the part of the mother, as she attempts to push her baby 'up hill'.

In 1965, Blankfield wrote:

If, in addition, the woman's back is lifted off the bed, further handicaps may be imposed upon her. Sometimes she is half somersaulted backwards and has to push against gravity as if she is about to launch a spaceman! . . . Frequently her head is unsupported and drops, so that she pushes into her throat. It is unreasonable to expect the patient to achieve this posture (flat back, thigh on abdomen) herself, as it requires exceptional muscular ability even under normal circumstances. Often, the patient is exhausted, and too tired even to grip her thighs – quite apart from raising her heavy torso and her floppy head.[13]

Also, the abdominal muscles which are trying to aid expulsion by raising the intra-abdominal pressure[14] have first to contract hard to attempt to bring the mother into a 'curved-back' position. If the mother does not give up the attempt in despair in the face of the overwhelming mechanical disadvantages, she is likely to find herself running out of time in hospitals where there is a time limit on the second stage. In both instances, the use of forceps or vacuum extraction is increased.

Increased traction when forceps are used

The obstetrician using forceps is faced with the same mechanical disadvantage as the mother if he tries to deliver a baby with the mother lying flat: the pull is horizontal and the baby's weight is vertical. Howard showed that if the mother is upright, only 80 per cent of the force needed in the horizontal position is needed to deliver the baby – the average pull exerted is 28 pounds, compared with 33.5 pounds for the horizontal position.[4]

Inhibition of placental delivery

In Newton's study it was found that the delivery of the placenta was quicker if the mother was sitting, and slower if she was lying down. If the spontaneous expulsion of the placenta is delayed, it is likely to be delivered by pulling on it, forcing it out by pushing on the uterus, or by manual removal (putting a hand inside the uterus and scraping it off the walls of the uterus with the fingers).[15, 16]

All these procedures increase the risk of foetal blood cells escaping into the mother's circulation,[17] although this is only significant if the mother is rhesus negative, or has ABO incompatibility. Finally, in the case of manual removal of the placenta, the mother is likely to bleed more, sometimes even to the extent of requiring a blood transfusion.

Low back strain

It is a prerequisite of placing a woman's feet in lithotomy poles that there be two assistants and that the legs be lifted together, as it is acknowledged that if the legs are lifted separately or unevenly low back discomfort or pain can arise from the rotatory strain imposed on the sacrum and lumbar vertebrae. However, the fact has often been overlooked that this strain can occur simply from overenthusiastic raising of the legs of the mother in labour by her attendants.[13]

Vaughan in 1937[18] presented X-rays and measurements which indicated that squatting alters pelvic shape in a way that is advantageous for delivery. More recently, Russell in 1969[19] showed radiographically that the cross-section surface area of the birth canal may increase dramatically, by as much as 30 per cent, when a woman changes from the dorsal to the squatting position. Less 'civilized' peoples have instinctively made use of this fact to overcome quite marked cephalo-pelvic disproportion. Numerous instances can be cited of women delivering themselves of still-born foetuses in situations where the degree of disproportion was such that their own lives were at risk from obstructed labour.[4] (In Western societies the problem of marked cephalo-pelvic disproportion would be resolved by Caesarean section.) If an attempt is made to rotate the squatting position through 90 degrees or more (the thigh-on-abdomen position, a variation of the lithotomy position), the result is less satisfactory, as the pelvis sways around in space instead of being anchored. This in turn prevents the muscles of the abdomen from contracting to their maximum advantage.

If the mother is lying flat, her legs are 'in the way' of the accoucheur, who is mainly interested in seeing the perineum. If the mother cannot hold them herself, then the alternative to putting the legs in lithotomy poles is for the attendants to hold them. The danger here is of imposing a sideways strain on the perineal tissues if the thighs are too far apart: this is discussed on page 142, as it involves the likelihood of tearing or episiotomy. An additional disadvantage to the mother arises if the attendants brace her feet against their hands (or very often their hips). It may be very convenient for the midwife if the mother's foot is on her hip, as she will then have both hands free, but the mother's instinctive reaction is to push against the brace with her flexed thighs. This is not only a waste of muscular effort, but it may also result in her pushing her body back up towards the head of the bed

It is not necessary for either the hands or the legs of the mother to be occupied when she is bearing down: much less extra energy is expended if she is allowed to let her legs flop in a semiflexed position, with her hands limply at her side.

A sitting or propped position requires some mechanical assistance if the mother is to be spared the considerable effort needed to flex herself. No less than 32 of the cultures studied by Naroll et al.[5] provided the mother with some means of support. Sometimes a stake is driven into the ground for her to hold on to: sometimes a rope suspended from ceiling or rafters to hang on to, or a post or wall against which to lean. Almost always they found that the mother was assisted by several female helpers – relatives, friends or midwives. Very commonly, some of this assistance was directly physically supportive – holding the mother from behind, or sitting her on a lap. In our Western hospitals, if the husband is not to be actively encouraged to join his wife on the delivery table to support her in his arms, then other means of support must be found. These may be provided in the form of cushions, pillows, beanbags or foam wedges placed against a wall or a back rest, or may take the form of a birth chair or a bed which adjusts to a chair-like position. The majority of mothers were found by Newton[9] to prefer an angle of inclination between 30–45 degrees, although some may wish to be even more upright than this. Properly supported, the woman has her spine curved in such a way as to allow her abdominal muscles to be used solely for their prime action of increasing the intra-abdominal pressure to aid expulsion of the baby.[20] Sitting, compared with seven other postures, was found by Mengert and Murphy to produce the greatest intra-abdominal pressure, due not only to the weight of the abdominal contents but also to increased muscular efficiency.

Only 65 per cent of the force necessary to effect delivery in the horizontal position is required if the mother sits up.[4, 14] Sitting up also allows the mother to bend her head forward slightly, so avoiding the uncomfortable feeling of pushing into her throat when she bears down.

In addition to the mechanical and physiological advantages of an upright position over a flat position, several psychological advantages are conferred. Mothers who are propped up for the second stage tend to take a more active and positive part in the delivery – the difference between 'doing' and 'being done to'. They are more able to cooperate with their attendants, and better able to see what is happening. They are more likely to show pleasure at the first sight of their babies (more frequently than those mothers who are flat for delivery), and are better able to hold them immediately after birth.[9]

A further argument, if one is needed, is the economic one. Just simply altering the mother's position – or more accurately, allowing her to choose it for herself – brings about a decreased need for analgesics, anaesthetics, surgical procedures such as episiotomy, perineal stitching, forceps or vacuum extraction, all of which add to the cost of a hospital delivery, and all of which will require the skills of a doctor who could be giving more of his time and attention to that minority of women who have problems which are not iatrogenic.

The exhortation to push

The conduct of the second stage in many Western hospitals is reminiscent of a rugby match: the all-too-familiar picture is one of a sweating, panting, pushing mother, being instructed to take a deep breath and hold it for as long as possible whilst bearing down, meanwhile surrounded by an expectant and enthusiastic audience exhorting her to further efforts. It is expected that she should be working very hard, getting very hot and red in the face, with her neck veins bulging. . . . Many of the onlookers will probably find that they are holding their breath in sympathy with the woman's exertions. Much cheering and encouragement accompanies each expulsive effort, and the atmosphere is tense and urgent, with the emphasis on 'aiding, abetting and even coercing the mother into forcing the foetus as fast as she can through the birth canal'.[21]

Suzanne Arms (author of *Immaculate Deception*) adds,

that mothers do not consciously remember the experience as silly and downright humiliating is due to their sincere efforts to please every one around them, and to the consuming effort of giving birth. . . . The team approach to childbirth . . . even if the delivery occurs without any form of analgesia or anaesthesia, is not to be confused with a natural birth, which can only take place in an atmosphere of calm and quiet faith. . . .[22]

The rationale for this insistence that the mother should hold her breath and strain is far from clear. It would appear that rather like the other nonphysiological traditions in obstetrics, it has been established by habit. There are several good reasons why this habit should be broken!

Taking a deep breath and holding it before attempting to push anything is uncomfortable and inefficient. No man would make an attempt to push a wardrobe by taking a deep breath – he might, however, hold his breath for brief periods, punctuated by a series of short grunts and groans. As long ago as 1965 Adele Blankfield wrote:

A misconception persists about inspiration in that the patient is told to take a deep breath and then push (Eastman, 1961; Brews, 1963). Negus (1929), together with Clayton, observed and measured the chest expansion of many subjects performing hard physical tasks and straining effort. . . . They noted that the chest was only slightly filled with air for these actions. They observed that it was most unusual for an initial deep breath to be taken. They concluded that maximal effort could be achieved with a small inspiration. It is extremely difficult to hold a deep breath for the following reasons: the lungs are elastic, and the more they are stretched, the greater the battle against their rebound recoil; . . . and the more the lungs are expanded, the more impulses arrive from higher centres demanding expiration.[24]

It is not necessary either, to 'fix the ribs and diaphragm' to achieve effective pressure when bearing down.[23]

The diaphragm is a sheet-like muscle which tires easily and is largely ineffective in sustaining a contraction when the breath is held.[25, 26] The technical name for the action described, of holding the breath and straining, is the Valsalva manoeuvre, so called after the seventeenth-century Italian doctor who first described it as a means of forcing pus out of the middle ear.

When the mother holds her breath, she seals off her windpipe by closing her giottis. If she then bears down, she raises the pressure in the chest cavity. If she maintains this pressure, she then dramatically reduces the blood flow back to the heart: the blood is dammed back in the venous system (hence the congestion in the mother's face) and the amount of oxygenated blood the heart can pump out is correspondingly reduced. In the meantime, the levels of carbon dioxide in her blood stream rise (as she is not breathing out) until she feels herself at bursting point, and is forced to gasp for a further breath. The sudden release of pressure in the chest is followed by a backlash or rebound rise in the previously low blood pressure. This sudden and high rise in blood pressure has been shown to cause alterations in heart-rate patterns (ECG), alterations in brain-wave patterns (EEG) and even strokes (CVA). While the woman is straining, the pressure in all the vessels and the cerebrospinal fluid is constant. It is during the release that damage may be done – burst capillaries are not uncommon in the faces and eyes of women straining in the second stage.

In addition to the far-reaching changes in the circulatory system, damage may also be done to the vagina, uterine supports, and skin and muscle of the perineum. First, slow, gentle distention of the vagina and perineum is much less likely to cause tearing than the rapid or sudden stretching which occurs if the baby's head is forced at speed down the birth canal by the manoeuvres described above[27] (see also pages 143–4). Secondly, if pushing begins simply because the mother is 'diagnosed' as being in the second stage rather than because she *wants* to push, then the baby is not simply being pushed down from above like a piston, as it would be if the head had reached the pelvic floor, but is actually causing the ring of contact with the vagina or even cervix to be dragged down, thereby pulling on the transverse cervical ligaments and connective tissue supports of the vagina.[21] Constance Beynon suggests that this may be a causative factor in uterovaginal prolapse.

Thirdly, if the woman is instructed to push from the very beginning of each contraction, the vagina does not have time to become taut, which it needs to be to prevent the anterior vaginal wall and the bladder with its supports from being pushed down in front of the baby's head. When this happens, a shearing strain is produced between the vaginal tissue and its deeper attachments. This may well be one of the factors in the development of stress incontinence later. Constance Beynon likened the process to a coat sleeve with a loose lining:

Firstly, the slower the arm is thrust down the sleeve, the less is the tendency for the lining to roll out at the wrist. Secondly, if the lining is held firmly at the top during the manoeuvre, the amount of resistance to the descending arm is considerably reduced, and its passage down the sleeve becomes much easier.[21]

As might be expected, the circulatory changes in the mother due to prolonged bearing down (i.e. longer than 5–7 seconds) will have a pronounced effect on the baby. If less blood gets back to the heart, then less blood leaves it, and there is a reduced blood flow to the placenta and therefore a drop in the amount of oxygen getting to the baby (foetal hypoxia). This is made worse as there is already a reduction of the amount of oxygen in the mother's blood.

Ironically, it is this foetal hypoxia . . . seen in the second stage of labour that is given as the reason why the second stage should be very short. It is recognized as being dangerous to the foetus, but it has not been understood until now that our instruction to the mother in the second stage to bear down long and hard is *causing* this foetal hypoxia. . . . Her *spontaneous* efforts are normally within physiological limits – about 5 or 6 seconds long.[28]

Dr Caldeyro-Barcia measured the strength and length of second-stage contractions and bearing-down efforts in mothers, and related them to simultaneous foetal heart-rate tracings. All bearing-down efforts produced at least a transient drop in the baby's heart rate as a result of head compression. Pushes lasting 5–6 seconds produced a quick recovery as the contraction finished, and no fall in heart rate after the contractions. When the push lasted 9 seconds, the heart rate fell to lower levels and remained low for longer. This he concluded was damaging, and pushes sustained for 15–18 seconds had a marked hypoxic effect on the baby.

There have been various articles on the subject of conservative second-stage management this century. As long ago as 1913, De Lee wrote,

The patient is not allowed to bear down overmuch during the first part of the second stage. The author does not hurry this period of labour without indication. . . . The levator ani and the fascia above and below it making up the pelvic diaphragm can only be spared serious injury by slow dilatation . . . with each pain the head is allowed to come down to distend the perineum a little more. . . .[29]

Jeffcoate in 1950 also made the point that it was better to begin expulsive efforts too late than too soon.[30] Beynon in 1957 added that it was better to strain too little than too much. When they are permitted to 'open up' to the messages coming from their uterus, and respond appropriately to them, most mothers do not need to be *told* when and how to push. But the character of the second-stage responses is likely to be different from the stereotyped labour-ward instructions. The urge to push comes at the height of the contraction, not at the beginning, and there is a clear interval between the onset of the contraction and the mother's urge to exert herself. Also, the amount of effort exerted involuntarily with each contraction will vary considerably. Some contractions may be short and mild, while others will be long and strong. There is no necessity for the mother to fix her diaphragm in order to use it, piston-like, on the uterus, as it is the abdominal muscles not the diaphragm which make the greatest contribution to the expulsive work of the uterus. Furthermore, these can only contract effectively as the mother breathes out (which is true of other forms of exercise and exertion): hence the grunting, which is often regarded with dismay as a 'waste of breath' by labour-ward staff, not only safeguards the mother and baby against the dangers of prolonged breath-holding, but also makes the voluntary pushing efforts more effective.[31, 32]

Some midwives take pride in conducting the second stage by encouraging and supporting the mother, if appropriate, without ever mentioning the word 'push', thus allowing the mother to follow her physiological inclinations. Those who have witnessed births handled in this way have been impressed by the ease of expulsion of the baby's head and the tranquil atmosphere that can be achieved.

Objections to the conduct of a delivery in this manner are likely to be based on a belief that the second stage will be prolonged, that the forceps rate will rise and that there may be danger to the baby from a long second stage. A clinical trial at Sussex Maternity Hospital has shown that these objections are unfounded.[21] Out of 100 mothers with no instructions given to them to push, only two second stages lasted more than two hours, and the forceps rate was half that of the control group. The need for stitches and/or episiotomy was moreover also half that of the control group. It is appropriate to recall here, too, the conclusion of Butler and his long-term study of 17,000 children (see page 136) that a second stage lasting as long as two and a half hours did not increase the incidence of neurological impairment in the full-term infant. A later study by Cohen (1977) also concluded that the practice of terminating labour after any arbitary time period in the second stage of labour could not be supported.[33]

Not all women have completely normal labours, and some will need additional guidance as to how best to coordinate their efforts. Some will need the assistance of forceps or vacuum extractor. Each labour is individual and must be considered on its merits and conducted appropriately, but it is surely reasonable to aim at giving every woman the chance to experience an unforced second stage by allowing her to synchronize her efforts with her own internal instructions, rather than those of the obstetrician or midwife with one eye on the clock. She will then be operating entirely within natural physiological limits, and will be more free also to achieve her own style of birth.

The use of fundal pressure to assist delivery of the baby

Fundal pressure – that is, pushing down on the top of the uterus in the direction of the vagina – is more commonly used as a method of delivering the placenta, and its use in this context is discussed in the section dealing with placental delivery. It is, however, still used by some as a method to speed delivery of the baby when there is 'delay' in the second stage.

Apart from being an inefficient 'aid' to delivery and causing intense pain to the mother, it has numerous other side effects:

1. It may bruise the abdominal and uterine walls.[34]

2. It may damage the bladder.[35]

3. It puts great strain on the uterine ligaments which support the uterus.[36, 37]

4. It impedes the placental circulation and reduces the amount of oxygen available to the baby.[38, 39, 40] Pennoyer has shown that there is a relationship between this reduction of oxygen due to the use of fundal pressure and clinically observed anoxia in the baby at birth.

The effects of fundal pressure are likely to be compounded by the situation in which it is used. Delay in the second stage is much more common where there are obstetric complications and when drugs with a sedative effect have been used. Unfortunately, these factors by themselves may diminish seriously the oxygen levels in the baby,[40] and pushing hard on the top of the uterus only serves to make the matter worse.

Consideration of the use of fundal pressure in the second stage is largely omitted from reputable obstetric textbooks, and ought similarly to be omitted from obstetric practice.

Episiotomy

Discussions on the subject of episiotomy are for most women heavily emotionally charged, and with good reason, as the performance of this surgical incision and more particularly its subsequent repair may crucially affect their future sexual wellbeing and self-image.

An episiotomy, which may be performed for a variety of reasons (see below), is a cut made in the perineum to enlarge the vaginal opening. The perineum or perineal body is made up principally by three of the various muscles which form the pelvic floor. This floor or 'sling' of pelvic muscles is responsible for the support of the pelvic organs (and indirectly the abdominal ones), controlling the passage of wind, faeces or urine, and for sexual response and satisfaction during intercourse. During the first stage of labour the normal muscle tone in the levator ani muscles (of which the puboccygeus muscle is part) ensures that direction and guidance is given to the baby's head as it descends – though this is removed if the mother has an epidural[41] – and during the normal and unhurried second stage, the muscles of the perineum thin out slowly and gently to allow the baby's head to be born. If the skin and muscle of the perineum and vagina do not have time to stretch sufficiently to allow the passage of the head, then tearing or laceration will result. These tears are usually classified as first-, second- and third-degree tears (1°, 2°, 3°), and are defined as 1° – superficial or skin tear, 2° – skin and muscle tear, and 3° – skin, muscle and anal sphincter tear. When an episiotomy is performed, skin and muscle are cut: it would seem logical, therefore, to use episiotomy as a means of preventing a third-degree tear or else controlling a possibly extensive second-degree tear.

There are three main types of episiotomy: midline, mediolateral and 'J'-shaped. They are usually performed with scis-

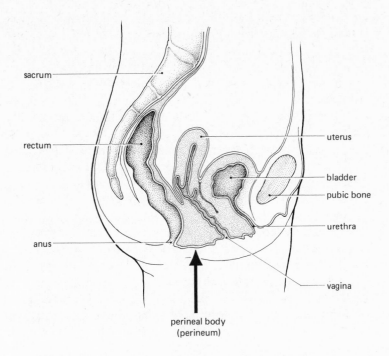

perineal body
(perineum)

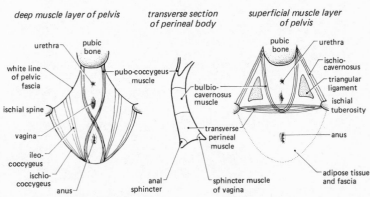

deep muscle layer of pelvis

transverse section
of perineal body

superficial muscle layer
of pelvis

sors. A midline incision enlarges the vaginal outlet in the way
that 'nature' is most likely to do it – by splitting the perineum
vertically in the midline towards the anus. This has several
advantages over the alternatives in that it bleeds less, is easier

to repair, less painful and less likely to cause pain on intercourse later. The main danger, and the reason it is not usually
used by midwives, is that if any extension of the incision takes
place during delivery, the anal sphincter is likely to be torn
– the very situation that the episiotomy was designed to
prevent.

A mediolateral incision starts in the midline and is then
directed diagonally to the right of the anal sphincter at about
7 o'clock (if the sphincter is considered to be 6 o'clock) and
is 3 – 4 cm long. This type of incision has the advantage of
protecting the anal sphincter, but it bleeds much more than
a midline incision and may cause vaginal tearing if it extends
during delivery. It is also more difficult to repair, heals more
slowly and is more likely to become infected. A 'J'-shaped
incision, performed with curved scissors, is a theoretical
compromise, as in practice it very often becomes mediolateral.
It starts in the midline and extends towards the anus for 1–2
cm, then curves away to the right. It has the advantage of
avoiding the anus and bleeding less than the mediolateral, but
suturing is difficult and the skin tends to pucker when
repaired.

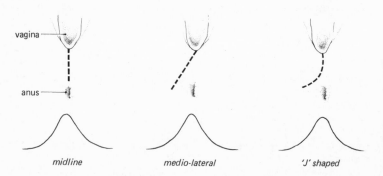

vagina

anus

midline   medio-lateral   'J' shaped

Historically, cutting the perineum in order to hasten delivery has been advocated sporadically: episiotomy procedure
was introduced in 1742 by Sir Fielding Ould,[42] the Irish
midwife, who cut the vulval outlet when it offered 'too great
resistance', and Michaelis in 1810 incised the perineum to

avoid a dangerous tear. However, a popular textbook of 1831 (Burns)[43] emphasized the importance of preserving the perineum, and discussed in detail labour-slowing techniques whereby this can be accomplished. In 1816, Merriman stated that

natural labour requires but little assistance on the part of the accoucheur. He must recollect that the dilatation of the soft parts will be effected by the natural pains, assisted by the bag of waters gradually insinuating itself through the uterus and vagina, much more easily and safely than by any artificial means that he can employ.[44]

The term 'episiotomy' was attributed to Braun in 1857, who condemned it as unadvisable and unnecessary.[45]

Midwives prior to 1967 were trained to prevent tears by conservative means, e.g. cooperation with the mother to ensure slow delivery of the baby's head and careful delivery of the shoulders. In June of that year the Central Midwives Board permitted midwives to perform episiotomy as an emergency measure, and today the indications for episiotomy and its technique are a standard part of a midwife's training. The list of indications for an episiotomy has grown so long in some hospitals that it is now a routine procedure, and in at least one hospital it is mandatory,[46] but the following are generally considered to be 'good' reasons:

1. Any situation which is likely to cause severe and/or third degree tearing, e.g. (a) baby in a face upwards position (persistent occipito-posterior position); (b) prior to a forcep delivery (and therefore in most hospitals prior to a breech delivery); (c) a previous third-degree tear (because scar tissue does not stretch well); (d) a perineum that does not stretch in response to the pressure of the baby's head and becomes white and shiny; (e) trickling of blood from the vagina when the baby's head is visible, which suggests that the vaginal tissue is beginning to tear; (f) a narrow pubic arch or android type of pelvis, which pushes the baby's head backwards onto the perineum.

2. When there is doubt about the baby's condition in the

second stage, an episiotomy will speed up the delivery and also facilitate the use of forceps if necessary.

3.   When the baby is premature, an episiotomy may prevent intracranial damage due to too rapid compression and decompression of the soft skull bones.

4.   When the mother's condition necessitates a short second stage with the minimum of pushing, e.g. severe pre-eclampsia or cardiac disease, or if the mother has ceased to make progress when the head is distending the perineum – as an alternative to a forceps delivery.

5.   Breech delivery – for the reasons given in (1) and also to prevent too rapid compression and decompression of the head which may not be 'soft' as is the case with a premature baby, but has, in the case of a breech birth to travel through the pelvis and vagina much more rapidly than is the case when a baby is born head first.

There are unfortunately a great many episiotomies performed for much less defensible reasons, as in the following instances.

1.   For a great many midwives an episiotomy has become 'respectable' where a tear or perineal laceration has not. So, to avoid the possibility of a first-degree or even a small second-degree tear, an episiotomy – equivalent in most cases to a large second-degree tear – is performed. In hospitals where even a small nick which requires no suturing is considered bad midwifery, then pupil midwives and medical students become so anxious lest the perineum tear that an episiotomy is the easiest solution. It is very rare to be criticized for an unnecessary episiotomy. This becomes a vicious circle, and the next generation of midwives and doctors will not know *how* to deliver a mother without an episiotomy, or even to judge the state of the perineum.

Furthermore, there is evidence to suggest that the increased use of episiotomy does not decrease the incidence of tears, and in a comparison between home and hospital deliveries, investigators found that despite a ninefold increase in the episiotomy rate for hospital over home deliveries, the hospital-delivered women still sustained a statistically and significantly greater number of first-, second- and third-degree tears.[47] This observation is confirmed by a study carried out in Cardiff (by Chalmers *et al.*) which showed that while the episiotomy rate doubled over the period 1965–73 (24.4 per cent to 46.7 per cent) the incidence of tears remained the same.[48]

2.   Although there were more trained staff available to look after fewer women in 1970 as compared with 1946, the proportion of women actually delivered by trained personnel has in fact decreased over this period.[49] Avoiding perineal lacerations and knowing whether an episiotomy is a better alternative to the tear which the midwife believes may be imminent are essentially matters of skill and judgement which come with experience. If, as has already been stated, tears are regarded as a mark of failure, then the inexperienced will perform an episiotomy whenever there is the slightest doubt about the perineum, or, what is even more likely, will be prevented from performing it only if the mother delivers her baby before there is time for the operation to be carried out.

3.   In a great many hospitals, there is an arbitrary time limit imposed on the second stage, of one to one and a half hours: after this time, the mother is subjected to an episiotomy and possibly also a forceps delivery, irrespective of the degree of progress she has made and the condition of the baby and/or herself. In some hospitals, notably in London, this time limit may be as little as half an hour – ludicrously short for the majority of first-time mothers.

This inability to sit quietly and let delivery take place gently and in its own time (assuming the mother and baby are well and that progress is being made) is justified by the statement that after this time the baby is at risk from possible oxygen shortage, or through the head's being compressed against the perineum. In fact, one obstetrician has said that for every minute the baby's head is on the perineum, two points can be deducted from its IQ![50]

There is no evidence to support any of these theories. The Director of the Centre for Birth and Human Development has added:

There does not seem to be any logical rationale for the image of the baby's head as a battering ram against the perineum, especially since in a normal birth the baby's head descends two steps forward and then ascends one step backwards, each time stretching the perineum more and more in a gradual process, rather than against the perineum.[51]

There has been a scientific study done of 17,000 children, all born during one week and followed up for seven years in Great Britain, which found no correlation between the length of the second stage of labour (up to two and a half hours) and the incidence of neurological impairment of the full-term infant who had showed no signs of foetal distress in labour.[52]

4.   The last major reason given for episiotomy, which 'justifies' 100 per cent episiotomy as a routine measure, is that all women have an inbuilt pelvic 'flaw' and if the midwife/obstetrician does not do them the kindness of cutting the perineum, there will be overstretching and damage to the pelvic supports, leading to prolapse in later life. Proponents of this argument will go on to suggest that if an episiotomy is *not* performed, then after the birth husbands will no longer be able to enjoy intercourse with their wives because the vagina will be permanently enlarged and misshapen. . . . Not only is there no evidence to support this theory, but there has recently been some research done in America which repudiates it. Mehl, Brandsel and Peterson compared two groups of women, one group of whom had delivered without episiotomy and the other group who had had episiotomies. The two groups were matched for age, race, parity, length of time since delivery, pattern of previous episiotomies, socioeconomic status, nursing status (whether they were breast-feeding) and pregnancy status (whether they were currently pregnant). They found no statistical difference between the

two groups with regard to the incidence of rectocele (weakening of the posterior wall of the vagina with protrusion of the rectum into the vagina), or with regard to muscle tone in the vagina and the ability to use the muscles to exert a squeezing action. They conclude that 'episiotomy is definitely *not* prophylactic against pelvic relaxation.'[51] House[53] also found that a search of the literature failed to find any evidence to support the claim that episiotomy could be justified on the grounds that it protected the mother.

Even when an episiotomy can be justified (by reference to the 'good' reasons) it still carries with it a number of side effects by comparison with perineal tears.

When tearing occurs, it takes place in most cases at the last possible moment just before the head crowns when the perineal tissue is stretched and thin. The timing of an episiotomy is for the most part in the hands of the accoucheur. If it is done too early when the perineum is still thick, then it will bleed profusely. An episiotomy that has been properly timed is likely to add about 153 ml (6 fl oz) to the total blood loss;[53] badly timed, an episiotomy may bleed so much that a blood transfusion becomes necessary.[46]

But much more commonly the tissues are crushed as they are cut. (The crush injury is worse still if the scissors are blunt.) Crushed tissues produce more bruising and swelling, and heal slowly, and this is likely to account for a fair proportion of those episiotomies which fail to heal spontaneously.

The same problem arises when the perineal tissues are liberally injected with local anaesthetic: they then become thick and spongy and also bleed more. The result of all this is more pain after delivery compared with that suffered by women who have not received local anaesthetic prior to episiotomy:[55] this is presumably because there is more crushing of the tissues. Normally, when tearing occurs it does so at the height of a contraction, when the baby's head is distending the perineum, and in this situation the tissues are under pressure and are numb. The tear, if perceived at all, is registered only as a feeling of giving way. If an episiotomy is performed without an anaesthetic, as it occasionally is, then it will be painless only if it mimics the tear and is done at the height of the contraction when the tissue is under pressure from the baby's head. If it is not, or if it is done with local anaesthetic which has not been given time to work, it is likely to be extremely painful.

Any woman who has an episiotomy performed obviously has to have it repaired: this necessitates her lying down flat with her feet in stirrups (the lithotomy position) which is at best a dreadful anticlimax after the excitement of having given birth, and at worst a humiliating and traumatic experience. The area to be stitched should always be anaesthetized, and it should never be assumed that the perineum and vagina are numb simply because delivery took place within a half-hour of the stitching, even though this may be true in some cases.

It is also indefensible to begin suturing until the anaesthetic is fully effective. To a woman who has just given birth, particularly if it was arduous, any pain after the delivery is more than she should be asked to tolerate. It is equally appalling that so little attention may be paid to the psychological wellbeing of the woman while her perineum is being sutured that she feels as though she is demeaned or sullied by the actions of the doctor. The mother needs to be sympathetically included in both procedure and conversation, not treated as though she were not present except from the waist downwards. . . .The situation might be improved if suturing of the perineum were included in the general training of the midwife, as it is in that of her European counterpart. This would seem a logical step to take since midwives now perform episiotomies: it would preserve the feeling of continuity (between mother and midwife) of delivering and stitching, and make it much less traumatic for the mother (to say nothing of reducing the number of times the GP or hospital resident gets out of bed 'just for stitches').

In addition to the problems of being badly cut, a great many women suffer because they have been badly stitched. 'The stitches were worse than having the baby' is an extremely common complaint amongst women, and a major factor in the comfort or otherwise of the perineum is the skill with which it is put back together. The muscles of the pelvic floor have to be accurately rejoined with absorbable stitches, sufficient to keep the muscle together and prevent blood from being collected in 'pockets' under the skin (haematoma) but not so many that there is no room for expansion caused by the inflammatory exudate which is part of the healing process and which puts the sutures under tension. It is also vital that the superficial tissues of the vagina and perineum (skin and mucosa) are correctly aligned and not stitched too tightly, otherwise great discomfort will be produced both as the perineum heals and when intercourse is resumed.[54] It would appear that keeping the skin closed by means of one continuous stitch under the skin entails less discomfort and produces quicker healing than the use of single stitches as large areas of tissue are not trapped under tension – which would increase as the skin began to heal. Also, nonabsorbable stitches which are put in too tightly are extremely painful to remove.

The advantage in the early postnatal period of using an absorbable Dexon stitch, which has been shown to cause less inflammatory reaction and therefore less swelling and wound tension, is unfortunately counterbalanced by the fact that it takes 60–90 days to be absorbed, and is likely to increase the incidence of pain on intercourse during this period, as the tissues are still being held by the material thus preventing painless stretching. It was the conclusion of a study by Buchan and Nicholls in 1980[56] that Dexon ought to be used in preference to silk, but that it should be removed on the fifth day following the delivery.

Apart from the pain a badly stitched perineum may cause, it is also more likely to 'break down' as a result of reducing the blood supply and become infected. This will then require frequent bathing with saline or Eusol to clean the area, dressings, heat lamps, ultraviolet therapy and eventually restitching. If the restitching is not undertaken, the perineum will slowly heal itself by granulation (filling in from the bottom up, rather than from the sides), and this will cause painful and abundant scar tissue.

The effects of pain due to the stitching of the vagina and perineum may be profound.

The fact that . . . they . . . have painful associations can have emotional repercussions and deeply affect a woman's capacity for sexual responsiveness. It is with the first attempts at intercourse after childbirth – whether or not it is successful from the man's point of view – that a pattern of anxiety, displeasure and even acute pain can be laid down which may persist long after the time when there is any obvious physical reason for apprehension or discomfort.[57]

This state of affairs is likely to put considerable strain on the marriage. It is of paramount importance that women who are still experiencing pain from their stitches ten to fourteen days after delivery do not wait for their postnatal examination, or longer, in the hope that 'it will get better by itself', but seek the aid of their general practitioner. The longer bad stitching is left, the more scar tissue forms, and the harder resuturing becomes: the woman may then be told that the repair should be delayed until she has another baby. In extreme cases, plastic surgery may be necessary.

It follows that the person undertaking the perineal repair carries considerable responsibility for the future physical and emotional wellbeing of the woman in question, and it should not be left in the hands of the inexperienced without supervision.

Episiotomies also appear to produce more scarring of the perineum than do tears, and more vaginal numbness.[47]

In extreme cases, deaths have been reported as a result of episiotomies which became infected. Between 1969 and 1977, three women died in one hospital in King County, Washington, USA, within ten days of giving birth, from infected episiotomy sites.[58] It would seem therefore that it is in the mother's interest to avoid any episiotomy if possible, and routine episiotomy at all costs. It is difficult to obtain statistical evidence on the episiotomy rates in our hospitals, but in England and Wales it was estimated to be 22.3 per cent in 1968 and 36.98 per cent in 1973.[59] If it were reasonable to assume that the increase had continued at the same rate, i.e. 3 per cent per year, then it would now (in 1982) be in the region of 66 per cent. However, if trends in London are anything to go by, this is a very conservative estimate: in 1977 the West Middlesex Hospital had a rate of 55 per cent, and by 1979 two other hospitals had a 90 per cent episiotomy rate.[46] By contrast, the episiotomy rate in Holland, which has not changed in recent years,[51, 60, 61] is around 8 per cent, while the incidence of pelvic relaxation or prolapse has dramatically declined – yet another argument against the prophylactic use of episiotomy to prevent overstretching.

A woman who is about to give birth is in no position to argue about whether an episiotomy is necessary in her case, and at that point she is obliged to trust the judgement of whoever is aiding her delivery. There are, however, several things which can be done by her, and ideally also by her partner, to reduce the likelihood of an episiotomy being performed.

1.   She can make sure it is recorded in her notes or verbally conveyed to the person delivering her that she wishes to avoid being cut if at all possible: this will then place the onus on the midwife/doctor to justify her/his action subsequently, should an episiotomy be performed, and hopefully it will reduce the likelihood of a routine incision.

2.   She should find a (mechanically) good position for the second stage. The position in which women most commonly find themselves for delivery is the lithotomy or supine position. Dr Caldeyro-Barcia has described this as 'the worst conceivable position for . . . delivery, short of being hanged by the feet!'[62] The same would be true also of episiotomy and its avoidance. If the woman is horizontal and pushing in the same plane, gravity as always is acting downwards, and the resultant force is being applied to the perineal tissues rather than, as it should be, to assist the baby in its journey down the vagina. If she sits up (or stands/squats/kneels on all fours) then gravity and the expulsive efforts are working together,

and the maximum pressure is being exerted in the same plane in which the baby is travelling.

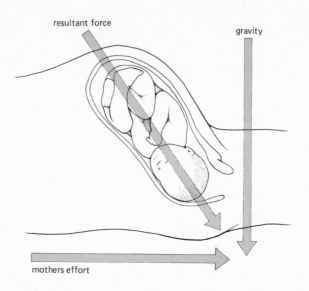

3.   The mother's knees should be about a foot apart to ensure that there is no sideways strain on the perineum. Again, with the very common lithotomy position, the feet are either placed in stirrups or held by an attendant: in both cases this nearly always results in the knees being held wide apart so that the perineum is already stressed before the baby's head begins to distend it, and what is more, stressed at right angles to the original tension. In this situation, tears and/or the apparent need for an episiotomy are very likely. In 1965 Blankfield (with reference to the work of Leak, 1955) wrote: 'The skin and fascia overlying the perineum are attached to the flexion creases of the thighs. Hyperflexion causes these tissues to become taut and drawn up so that the introitus is narrowed; this can predispose to tears.'[63] The mother should either keep her feet rolled with the soles inwards, and resting on the bed with her legs flexed slightly, or she may raise her legs and feet by placing her hands round or under her knees. If the woman

is permitted to position her legs herself, she is unlikely to choose a position which strains her perineum.

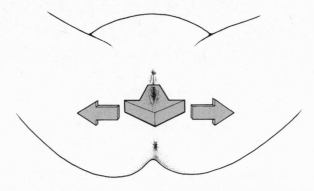

4.   In the antenatal period the performance of pelvic-floor exercises is of great benefit in preparing the mother for her second stage.[51, 64, 65] If she understands and has control of her pelvic floor muscles, she can respond appropriately to the sensations of the second stage and the midwife's instructions, and is far more likely to emerge unscathed from the delivery. Most antenatal teachers and books on preparation for childbirth have their own favourite approaches when it comes to teaching pelvic-floor control, such as stopping and starting a urine stream, slowly tightening and relaxing the anal sphincter to learn differentiation and control, but the one which is generally considered to be the most useful is the 'lift shaft' or 'invisible lift' exercise, when the woman is asked to imagine her pelvic floor as a lift which is slowly pulled up to four, five (or six!) floors, and then allowed to descend slowly and is finally 'bulged out' to allow the lift to enter the basement. This 'bulging' is what has to happen in the second stage to allow the head to be born, and familiarity with the sensations of pelvic-floor contraction will mean that the woman will recognize the feeling if she starts to tighten up in the second stage – so that instruction to relax her muscles or allow herself to open up will have much more meaning. Her rapport and her ability to cooperate with the midwife/doctor and achieve a gentle and unhurried second stage allowing the uterine con-

tractions and involuntary expulsive efforts alone to push the head down on to the perineum – all this will give the perineal muscles time to thin out and stretch. When the baby's head is about to be born, good pelvic-floor control will enable the mother to 'breathe the head out' slowly, rather than forcing it out rapidly – the latter being much more likely to result in perineal tears.

5.   If the mother has had an epidural during the first stage of labour, and it remains effective during the second stage, the incidence of forceps delivery and therefore episiotomy is greatly increased.[41] If matters can be so managed, however, that the epidural wears off during the second stage, then pushing is likely to be more effective and the need for instrumental delivery reduced.[41]

Naturally, any mother would like to give birth with her perineum intact. However, if an episiotomy is truly necessary and the mother and her partner can appreciate the reason for it, then, provided that it is properly performed and carefully repaired so that she feels afterwards that she is as she was before, the procedure should be one that most mothers can come to terms with. 'What is wrong with the practice of episiotomy at present is not episiotomy itself, but that it has become a mere obstetric fashion, and therefore a questionable routine.'[46]

Chapter 7

The third stage

The routine use of ergometrine and syntometrine

The use of ergometrine and more recently syntometrine in the management of the third stage of labour (from the birth of the baby to delivery of the placenta) was the response of obstetricians to the problems of postpartum haemorrhage, that is, blood lost after the birth of the baby (amounting to 500 ml–20 fl oz in volume) and 'As so often with developments in obstetrics [in most hospitals] all mothers came to be treated in the same manner, irrespective of the degree of risk [of their bleeding]'.[1]

It has been suggested that the prevalence of postpartum haemorrhage (PPH) in Western society is to an extent a 'man-made' problem. Botha[2] has pointed out that despite detailed biblical references to childbirth, menstruation and menorrhagia, there are no references to retained placenta or PPH. He adds, 'Since the sixteenth century much has been written about the third stage of labour; its management seems to present a bigger problem to us than to primitive peoples.' He then goes on to describe a Bantu birth in which the woman delivers her baby in a squatting position, and remains in the same position while the placenta delivers itself by gravity.

The mother then lifts herself onto her haunches and the membranes fall out. Only when the placenta is completely delivered does she pay any attention to the cord. He continues, 'Working among the Bantu for ten years, attending 26,000 Bantu and seeing only abnormal cases, I found many other complications, but a retained placenta was seldom seen. . . .' 'Blood transfusion for postpartum haemorrhage was never necessary.'

In contrast, postpartum haemorrhage (and retained placenta) was responsible for 14 per cent of maternal deaths in England and Wales up until 1976, when it fell to 9.2 per cent. (In 1919, 450 mothers died and in 1971, 19 mothers.)[3] The commonest cause of PPH is a failure of the uterus to contract and control bleeding from the placental site. This may be due to a number of reasons, amongst which are: twin pregnancy, prolonged or precipitate labour, a lax uterus as a result of repeated pregnancies, the administration of large doses of sedative drugs or deep anaesthesia. There are also circumstances where the uterus is unable to contract properly, either because there is something inside, e.g. partially separated placenta, retained portions of placenta or membrane, large fibroids, or else blood in the muscle wall of the uterus as a result of a severe bleed just before the onset of labour (antepartum haemorrhage), which makes the wall stiff and inelastic. Occasionally mismanagement of the third stage by the attendant is responsible for inefficient contraction of the uterus, e.g. allowing the woman to enter the third stage with a full bladder, or meddling with the uterus ('fundal fiddling') which may cause irregular contractions and partial separation of the placenta. Other major causes of postpartum haemorrhage are tissue damage – that is, episiotomies, vaginal, cervical or perineal tears, and coagulation disorders, i.e. a failure of the blood to clot. With regard to tissue damage, a study done by Paull and Ratten showed that the PPH rate among the women in their sample who required perineal stitches was 7 per cent, and if the perineum remained intact, the rate was 1 per cent.[4]

The use of syntometrine and ergometrine is likely to affect

only haemorrhage which is caused by the uterus failing to contract. Syntometrine contains 5 units of oxytocin (Syntocinon) and 0.5 mg of ergometrine.

Ergot

Ergot is a fungal infection of rye and its effect on the uterus has been known for centuries.[5, 6] It was first written about by Adam Loncier in 1582, and European midwives used it throughout the seventeenth and eighteenth centuries. However, in its crude form it could be extremely dangerous, and this tended to limit its usage. Its ability to induce 'St Anthony's fire' (a burning feeling in the hands and feet and reddened face caused by spasm of the blood vessels which often led ultimately to gangrene) was well known.[7]

In 1807 John Stearns of New York State reintroduced the substance but failed to generate much enthusiasm. In 1808 he sent a letter to a colleague (which was subsequently published in a medical journal) describing how he had been 'importuned' by a local midwife to search in granaries for the diseased heads of rye and to administer them in a decoction to women whose labours were abnormally slow,[8] and the letter went on to describe the remarkable effect of ergot.

This letter (and others) by Dr John Stearn was 'rediscovered' in 1932 by Dr J. Chassar Moir and he initiated the modern revival of ergot in obstetrics. Ergotoxine (1906) and ergotamine (1918) had already been isolated from ergot, but in 1935 simultaneous announcements of the isolation of a new water-soluble ergot principle came from Baltimore, Chicago, Basle, and London (Moir and Dudley). All the substances were found to be identical but they all had different names – ergonovine and ergotrate (USA), ergobasine (Switzerland), and ergometrine (UK). This newly discovered substance could be given by intramuscular or intravenous injection and was thought to be free of dangerous side effects. It was, however, noted to cause the placenta to be trapped within the uterus if given before the delivery of the placenta (retained placenta).[9]

Oxytocin

Natural oxytocin is produced by the pituitary gland: this gland is situated at the base of the brain and has two parts, front (anterior) and back (posterior). In the female, the front portion produces (amongst others) the milk-stimulating hormone (prolactin), and the back portion produces (amongst others) natural oxytocin, which stimulates the uterus to contract during labour. At the turn of the century, researchers investigating the effect of pituitary gland extract on the blood pressure of a cat discovered that it had the unexpected property of causing instantaneous and intense contraction of the uterus. Moir, in recounting its history, remarks that it was fortunate for medical science that the experimental animal was a tabby and not a tom![8] Unfortunately the early use of the extract was beset with difficulties, as the strengths of the commercial preparations were very uncertain, and varied dramatically: despite standardization in the early 1930s, the response in individual women remained unpredictable. By 1948 a new method of administration was introduced, the slow intravenous infusion of a very dilute solution of the drug – the now well-known oxytocin 'drip'.

A pure form of pituitary extract was developed by Du Vigneaud in 1954, synthesized by Boissonnas shortly afterwards and marketed under the name of Syntocinon.

Given *intravenously*, Syntocinon is effective in making the uterus contract in 40 seconds; *intramuscularly*, it takes $2\frac{1}{2}$ minutes.

Given *intravenously*, ergometrine is effective in making the uterus contract in 40 seconds; *intramuscularly*, it takes 6–7 minutes. With ergometrine, in particular, the dosage is important: for intramuscular use 0.5 mg is recommended and for intravenous use 0.25 mg (half the intramuscular dose). They act on different parts of the uterus, causing the muscle to contract. 'Oxytocin (Syntocinon) induces strong rhythmic uterine contractions . . . by affecting primarily the upper uterine segment. . . . Ergometrine induces unphysiologic uterine spasm . . . and affects the lower uterine segment'[10] (and cervix).

The newly discovered ergometrine had to be given intravenously if it was to be effective in stopping or preventing haemorrhage, as 6–7 minutes was far too long to wait in the face of a heavy postpartum bleed. In the early 1960s, workers at University College Hospital in London realized that pulling on the cord to deliver the placenta reduced the incidence of retained placenta if ergometrine were given before its delivery.

So the practice of administering intravenous ergometrine with the anterior shoulder of the baby (the first shoulder born) became widespread. The alternative, also developed in the early 1960s, was syntometrine: this mixture (5 units of Syntocinon and 0.5 mg ergometrine) was administered intramuscularly with the birth of the anterior shoulder, prior to delivery of the placenta by pulling on the cord. This alternative was principally for use by midwives who were not usually trained to give intravenous drugs. (Prior to this midwives had been using ergometrine which they mixed with hyaluronidase in an attempt to speed the action of IM ergometrine. This was unsatisfactory as the two substances had to be kept in separate ampules and only mixed just prior to administration.)

The practice of 'actively managing' the third stage quickly spread, and discussions revolved around which drug was best; when to give it (with crowning of the head, with the anterior shoulder, after the birth of the baby, or after delivery of the placenta); how to give it (intravenously or intramuscularly); and how to deliver the placenta having given an oxytocic drug, i.e. pulling on the cord (controlled cord traction or CCT), maternal effort, or fundal pressure (pushing downwards on the uterus). Many papers were published comparing the effectiveness of the two drugs, the alternative routes of administration and the methods of placental delivery. With the introduction of ergometrine and syntometrine the PPH rate fell, and undoubtedly a great many lives were saved by their use. Postpartum haemorrhage is a terrifying event for mother, midwife and obstetrician alike, and the discovery and application of these oxytocic drugs stands as one of the 'enduring achievements of modern science'.[8]

However, the use of these drugs rapidly became routine 'prophylaxis' for all women, irrespective of the degree of risk, and few workers actually studied the use of oxytocic drugs with a comparison using a nontreated control group of mothers.

Ergometrine, particularly when given intravenously, has unpleasant and occasionally dangerous side effects, probably due to its indiscriminate action on smooth muscle, including the heart and blood vessels. Headache, dizziness, ringing in the ears, chest pain, palpitations and cramplike pain in the back and legs have been reported.[11] Nausea and vomiting (which may occur to a mild extent following delivery where no oxytocic drugs are used) is made worse by the use of ergometrine: 4.5 per cent in a control group and 19.5 per cent in an ergometrine group was reported by Friedman[12] who in his study also found intractable nausea and vomiting in 2 per cent of the mothers who received ergometrine, and none in the control group.

Work done by the Department of Anaesthetics in Manchester[13] suggests that intravenous ergometrine given to women who have been delivered under anaesthesia may occasionally predispose to the development of acute pulmonary or cerebral oedema after delivery (engorgement or congestion of the lungs or brain with fluid from the circulatory system, causing severe breathlessness in the case of the lungs, and, in the case of the brain, headaches, vomiting, blurring of the vision and in severe cases increased drowsiness and eventual coma).

The most common serious effect is that which ergometrine has on the blood pressure. Much research has shown that ergometrine can produce a sharp rise in blood pressure in susceptible women which would appear to correspond to 12 per cent of subjects[9] – Forman and Sullivan in 1952, Friedman in 1957, Ringrose in 1962, Howard in 1964, Browning in 1974, and Hacker and Biggs in 1979.[11-16] This figure may be a conservative estimate, as it has been shown that if blood pressure is monitored continuously, rises of 20 mmHg may occur without symptoms.[17] 'Minor and even moderate degrees of blood pressure may be much more common than we realize.'[11]

Even a moderate rise in blood pressure may be dangerous in women who already have high blood pressure or toxaemia (pre-eclampsia).[9, 11] Several instances of the development of very high blood pressure with accompanying severe frontal headaches have been documented[11, 14] and having a fit as a result of the sudden elevation in blood pressure (eclampsia) has occurred in some cases as a result of ergometrine administration.[9, 11] There have also been reported instances of cardiac arrest[11, 18] and at least one death due to the effects of high blood pressure; there were more deaths due to uterine rupture following the routine administration of syntometrine before it was discovered that there was difficulty in delivering the baby's shoulders.[19]

There are other drawbacks associated with the use of ergometrine and syntometrine.

1. The midwife (or obstetrician) has to decide between clamping the cord immediately the baby is born, thereby denying it its extra physiological quota of 90 ml (3 oz) of blood;[20] or alternatively leaving the cord and risking the possibility of the baby becoming overtransfused as blood is forced into the baby by the energetic contractions of the uterus.

In 1960 Montgomery wrote.

Unfavourable also is the practice of administering intravenous ergotrate immediately upon the birth of the anterior shoulder of the newborn. This unphysiological procedure necessitates a choice between immediate clamping of the cord upon the birth of the newborn, or submitting the foetal circulation to a large quantity of blood forced over from the placenta by the vigorous contraction of the uterus and the influence of IV ergotrate. All this is over and above the unfavourable effect IV ergotrate may have on the circulation of the mother.[21]

It has also been suggested that this process of overtransfusion may begin in utero, as the placenta is squeezed like a sponge (following the administration of oxytocic agents), and that this may be the main reason for the rise in the number of newborn babies with so-called 'physiological jaundice' severe enough to cause anxiety to paediatricians. An investigation was begun in 1980 at the Horton General Hospital, Banbury, in an attempt to clarify this issue.[22]

There is evidence that clamping the cord immediately predisposes to transplacental haemorrhage,[23] and increased incidence of maternal bleeding[24] due to interference with the mechanisms of placental separation[2] (see pages 162–3). Ergometrine itself interferes with the physiology of placental separation by inducing an 'unphysiologic uterine spasm . . . which may result in partial retention of the placenta. This carries a higher risk of heavy bleeding and . . . general anaesthetic for manual removal.'[10]

2.   The midwife is rushed into getting the placenta out before the ergometrine (given intramuscularly as syntometrine) starts to work (seven minutes), and this inevitably means interfering with the mother's response to her newborn baby. She must interrupt their first moments of meeting one another to ask the mother to push out the placenta, or more commonly the midwife will pull it out herself by the cord, with her other hand on the mother's abdomen 'guarding' the uterus (see page 174). If the delivery of the placenta is delayed and the ergometrine is given time to come into action, the placenta may be trapped as the circular muscle fibres at the lower part of the uterus and cervix contract. In this situation, the spasm must be relieved either by giving the mother amyl nitrite to inhale which relaxes smooth muscle (and will make the mother feel very flushed for a few moments as the blood vessels also 'relax' – precisely the state of affairs that the ergometrine was given to prevent!), or by administration of a general anaesthetic, followed by *manual* removal of the placenta.

The combination of these two factors (partial separation or trapping of the placenta) means that the incidence of general anaesthetic for manual removal of the placenta is increased[25–28] where ergometrine is used. This, as Professor Dewhurst remarks, may not be too big a price to pay for preventing excessive blood loss when the women are at 'high risk', having previously had problems in the third stage of labour – as was the case in his study – but it is open to question whether the routine, prophylactic use of ergometrine (on its own or as syntometrine) is justified in cases where there is no anticipated problem if it increases the likelihood of a general anaesthetic, itself a potential cause of maternal death.

A further problem encountered with the routine use of ergometrine in some form prior to the delivery of the baby is that of trapping the undiagnosed second twin or third triplet. Undiagnosed 'extra' babies are not common, and a large maternity hospital might expect one or two per year – for example, the Royal Women's Hospital in Melbourne had eight cases between 1970 and 1977.[29] But there is a high mortality rate (35 per cent) and a high incidence of brain damage in babies which do survive the devastating effect of having ergometrine administered to the mother whilst they are still in utero.[29] This might be considered an argument against a routine oxytocic in low-risk women, at least before the baby is completely born and the presence of an unexpected sibling has therefore been excluded.

Apparently the fear of haemorrhage has meant that, since the isolation and widespread use of ergometrine and oxytocin, most investigations of the use of drugs in the management of the third stage of labour have been restricted to a comparison of specific oxytocic drugs, without the benefit of a nontreated control group as a base line. However, the few studies which have included a control (placebo) group have yielded some interesting information. Howard *et al.* in 1964 studied 1500 women divided into three groups, one of which was given oxytocin, one an ergot derivative, and one salt water. In each case, neither the mother nor her attendant knew which 'drug' was being given, and in each case the drug was administered after the delivery of the placenta. They found that there was no significant difference in the blood loss between the three groups in mothers who lost less than 500 ml (approximately one pint) but that there was among mothers who lost more than 500 ml – 3.2 per cent of the oxytocin group, 1.8 per cent of the ergometrine group, 5.3 per cent of the placebo group. They concluded that since 5 per cent of the mothers in the oxytocin and in the ergot group still needed further treatment (because the uterus failed to contract properly) and 12 per cent of the mothers in the placebo group needed further treatment (this figure falls to 10 per cent if the mothers who needed uterine massage only are excluded), then the routine use of oxytocic drugs *benefited only seven women in every 100*. The influence on blood pressure revealed by this study has already been referred to: significant increases in blood pressure in women whose blood pressure had been normal prior to delivery were recorded in 47 per cent of the ergot group, 38 per cent of the oxytocin group, and 31 per cent of the placebo group. In women who had already high blood pressure, the increases were 30.7 per cent of the ergot group, 11.5 per cent of the oxytocin group, and 7.9 per cent of the placebo group.[15]

Newton *et al.* (1961) compared two groups of 50 women, one group receiving oxytocin routinely after the delivery of the placenta, and the other not. They found no significant difference between the two groups in the amount of blood lost during delivery and in the first hour after delivery, although more of the control group required additional treatment.[30] (There were no notable changes in blood pressure in either group.)

Hacker and Biggs[16] compared three small groups who received intravenous ergometrine, intramuscular syntometrine and nothing, respectively, twenty minutes after delivery of the baby (and placenta). No other drugs were given to any woman during the recording period, in any group, and they found a postpartum blood loss of less than 200 mls (approximately 8 fl. oz) *in each mother*. However, despite the fact that all the mothers in the study had normal blood pressure to start with, *all* the mothers in the ergometrine group and 60 per cent in the syntometrine group had moderate to severe increases in blood pressure, whilst there were no moderate to severe increases in the control group.[16]

Friedman compared five groups, of whom the first received

nothing, the second oxytocin intramuscularly, and the other three each received one of three different kinds of ergot derivative, all administered after delivery of the placenta. His conclusion was 'that the proper management of the fourth stage of labour (the first hour after delivery) did not require routine use of an oxytocic agent was illustrated in the control group of patients, 78 per cent of whom did quite well without medication'. (This figure is similar to Newton's.) Of the 22 per cent who did require treatment, a proportion (unspecified) responded to uterine massage without the use of oxytocic drugs. He also found a statistically significant increase in the incidence of nausea and vomiting and of high blood pressure following the use of ergot derivatives.[12] It has also been shown that oxytocin is as effective as ergot preparations in preventing PPH and does not have the same severe side effects.[31]

Clarke and Douglas[32] compared the use of ergometrine and oxytocin singly and in combination with a control group. All the mothers in the trial, except the primigravidae (mothers having their first babies), were at high risk by virtue of bad obstetric history, emergency admission, toxaemia, anaemia or grand multiparity (seven pregnancies or more). The only mothers excluded from the randomized trial were those who had previously had third-stage difficulties, PPH or retained placenta, as it was thought dangerous to use mothers in this category as inert controls. Even in this study it was found that 60 per cent of women in the control group 'had efficient uterine action and were in no danger of haemorrhage'.

Sorbe[10] (1978) compared three groups, receiving intravenous ergometrine, intravenous oxytocin and nothing, respectively. He found that the ergometrine group had significantly more retained placenta than the other two, and as a result, the PPH was lower in the oxytocin group compared with the other two groups. He also found that 80 per cent of the control group had a blood loss of less than 500 ml (1 pt) compared with 88 per cent in the ergometrine group and 90 per cent in the oxytocin group. He concluded that when an oxytocic drug *was* required oxytocin given intravenously in adequate doses (in this study 10 units) reduced the PPH rate without interfering with the physiological mechanism of placental separation. This result confirmed work by Finnish researchers in 1964, who compared syntometrine with oxytocin (Syntocinon) and found that the PPH rate was the same in both groups (even though the third stage took longer to complete in the oxytocin group), but that the incidence of retained placenta was greater with syntometrine.[33]

There is no doubt that at the time when ergot was reintroduced postpartum haemorrhage was responsible for the deaths of hundreds of women a year, and that subsequently ergometrine has prevented a great many deaths as well as preventing significant haemorrhage in women who started to bleed. However, ergometrine is not the only factor which can possibly be related to the drop in the number of deaths from PPH. Since 1932, more women at risk from third-stage complications have been confined in hospital, the 'fourth stage of labour'[34] has been recognized as potentially hazardous, and closer watch has been kept on women for the first hour after delivery. Blood banks and blood transfusion services are available, as are 'flying squad' facilities. Deaths due to secondary PPH (i.e. occurring after twenty-four hours) have been reduced by the wider availability of good anaesthetics and surgical techniques (to remove retained placental fragments) and antibiotics have reduced deaths from secondary PPH due to infection of these retained fragments. Additionally, a pure synthetic form of oxytocin has been developed which has a more physiological action on the uterus than ergometrine.

There may now be sufficient evidence to suggest that the *routine* use of ergometrine should be abandoned altogether, and that it should be used only in selected high-risk situations. Ringrose,[14] in discussing the death of a seventeen-year-old girl who had had a normal pregnancy, labour and delivery, stated, 'It is likely that blind adherence to the postpartum ritual was contributory or causative in this death [from intercranial haemorrhage]. It is possible that the prophylactic use of ergot is . . . fraught with danger and not to be condoned unless definite indications are present.'

In view of the dangers associated with the prophylatic use

of any oxytocic drug (oxytocin or ergometrine) why is it still being used for women who are not considered to be at risk? 'Those women who have a normal first and second stage could be allowed to complete the process normally.'[1] This would then allow the mother (unhurried by the midwife since there would be no urgency to deliver the placenta within seven minutes) to experience the full tide of emotional feelings which themselves would stimulate the release of *natural* oxytocin with its contracting effect on the uterus.[35] The baby who is interested in sucking straight away can also be put to the breast, causing the release of yet more natural oxytocin. Since there would be no risk of overtransfusion for the normal infant, the cord can be allowed to finish pulsating before being divided, and this would allow rapid physiological separation of the placenta and reduce the blood loss still further.[36] (See also pages 161–2.)

Again, while the third stage is progressing normally, there is no reason to hurry delivery of the placenta by pushing on the uterus or pulling on the cord, and the mother should be allowed to expel it herself, making use of the effects of gravity.

A potential objection to the abandonment of routine oxytocics in the management of the third stage, even with 'low-risk' women, is the difficulty of predicting which women make up the 10–20 per cent who would bleed if untreated. Several factors have been suggested by various researchers as predisposing to postpartum haemorrhage. (Apart from previous third-stage problems, twins, placenta praevia, antepartum haemorrhage due to partial separation of the placenta (abruption), or anaemia – all of which would probably be known before the onset of labour.) For instance, prolonged first or second stage, poor second-stage contractions, or a precipitate labour: and the presence of these factors might alert the mother's attendants to the possibility of bleeding and the original decision – to withhold prophylactic oxytocics – could be reversed. In other words, a potentially low-risk situation could be treated individually, on its merits.

It should also be noted that with the unplanned use of oxytocics in the case of 12 per cent of the unselected control group[15] who started to bleed, only 5 per cent lost more than 500 mls (i.e. had a PPH) and that in the case of the other two oxytocic groups, 5 per cent of mothers had uteri that failed to contract properly, thereby necessitating further treatment, in spite of receiving prophylactic drugs. Further, as was pointed out at the beginning of this section, postpartum haemorrhages are not 100 per cent preventable even if oxytocic drugs are used prophylactically for all mothers, as these PPH may be due to causes other than uterine atony (failure of the uterus to contract).

A midwife attending a low-risk mother who suddenly bleeds would be in the *same* position, in the absence of routine administration of syntometrine, as she is now. Syntometrine takes two and a half minutes to work if given intramuscularly, and a great deal of blood can be lost in two and a half minutes from a uterus which fails to contract. The giving of intravenous injections is not normally within the province of the midwife any more than taking blood samples would be; but midwives in common with, for instance, anaesthetic nurses, can and do take blood samples with the approval of the institution in which they work, provided they have received instruction and are adjudged to be proficient. The same could apply equally to intravenous injections by midwives working in hospitals, and could also be incorporated into midwives' training. At present, midwives working on their own in domiciliary practice will give intravenous injections 'on behalf of the doctor' if an emergency situation demands it. It is illogical to ask midwives to give intramuscular syntometrine to *all* women on the grounds that they 'cannot' give intravenous injections to the few who may require them, when all that is necessary is extra tuition for the midwives.

As long ago as 1966, J. H. Patterson[37] expressed the view that ergometrine should be avoided before the birth of the baby, and only used before completion of the third stage in cases with significant bleeding; that *oxytocin* (Syntocinon) rather than ergometrine should be given in cases with a history of PPH or other special circumstances, and that cord traction (pulling on the cord) should be tried for removal of the undescended placenta *only* when bleeding indicates immediate action, or if after thirty minutes the natural process has not occurred. This should be backed up by manual removal if cord traction fails. Clarke and Douglas[32] had earlier maintained that in high-risk cases oxytocin should be given alone with the anterior shoulder (intramuscularly) and that ergometrine should be given intramuscularly only after placental delivery. If bleeding occurs and intravenous ergometrine is necessary, Paull and Ratten's research[4] has shown that the administration of 0.25 mg was associated with fewer side effects (without affecting the incidence of PPH or manual removal later) than the dosage of 0.5 mg, which is currently employed in most hospitals. (This despite the fact that Moir himself recommended that the intravenous dose should not exceed 0.25 mg.)[38]

There has been very little research to reassess the management of the third stage undertaken in the last fifteen years. Practices vary from country to country, and from hospital to hospital within a country, and up-to-date, randomized, controlled studies are urgently needed to clarify the situation. At present, such evidence as does exist calls into question the current practice of using routine oxytocics, particularly ergometrine, in the management of the third stage.

The umbilical cord

In the sections considering the positions which might be adopted by the labouring woman for the first and second stages of labour, it has been seen that over 80 per cent of 'primitive' people will adopt some variation of an upright position. As a consequence of this, the baby when born would be placed between the mother's legs initially, while the mother delivered herself of the placenta (in the manner described in the previous section). If she were adopting a sitting position, the baby might be brought up onto her abdomen for her to hold or she might even lean forward and put it to the breast. In both instances, the baby would be approximately at or below the level of the placental site for the time it would take the cord to stop pulsating. It is also the practice of the vast majority of these peoples to delay the cutting of the cord for an average of fifteen to twenty minutes *after the delivery of the placenta*.[39, 40] (In instances where the cord is cut before delivery of the placenta there is dependence on the invention of methods to staunch the extra bleeding which results.) In many cultures there are delays of several hours before the cord is cut. Commenting on her investigations, Margaret Mead notes:

The Manus of the Admiralty Islands place the crying neonate, cord uncut, facing the mother, in the belief that sight and sound together will facilitate delivery of the placenta. This raises the question of whether the sight of the neonate as well as the sound of its crying is involved in a biological releasing mechanism which should be taken into account in planning delivery style.[41]

It would certainly seem that the normal physiological process involves delivery of both baby and placenta before anything happens to the cord. A woman giving birth unaided is not likely to have anything about her with which to sever the cord, and she could not easily transport herself and her baby while the placenta was still in the uterus, even assuming she shared the urgency of many midwives and obstetricians to separate the baby from its placenta as quickly as possible. (Dr de Courcy-Wheeler wrote, 'This practice (of leaving the cord to finish pulsating) appears to have gone into abeyance in a number of places – due no doubt to the haste in producing the babies and getting on with the next case!'[42]

It seems intuitively likely that the physiological process has evolved for some good reason, and that in the majority of cases it cannot be improved upon. Any interference with the natural order of things is likely (with few exceptions) to be detrimental to mother, child or both. However, as might be expected, the third stage of labour has not escaped Western influence. In the mid-seventeenth century, as more and more men entered the field of midwifery, cord clamping became the rule, and for no better reasons than that the bed linen was spared if the maternal end of the cord was clamped, and it was also easier to tell when the cord lengthened – indicating that the placenta had separated and descended into the lower portion of the uterus.[43] Despite warnings that this practice might be harmful – Erasmus Darwin in 1803 wrote 'Another thing very injurious to the child is the tying and cutting of the navel string too soon',[44] and Meadows in 1881 referred in his manual of midwifery to Dewee's observation that the uterus contracted better and facilitated the expulsion of the placenta if the maternal side was not clamped[45] – despite all this the practice has continued to the present day, and it is very likely that it has contributed to the deaths of many women as a result of postpartum haemorrhage by interfering with the physiology of placental separation.

As the baby is born the contracting uterus rapidly reduces its own size and that of the placental site by a process of contraction and retraction of the muscle fibres in the uterus (retraction is the progressive shortening and 'fattening' of the muscle fibres as it contracts and relaxes). This process has been taking place throughout labour, and assists the dilation of the cervix and expulsion of the baby. The placenta does not separate during the normal first and second stages as the placental site has to be reduced by approximately half its original size before separation begins. Once the baby is being born, the uterus can reduce itself sufficiently for the process of separation to begin. As the placental site is reduced, the placenta itself is squeezed, and the blood in the spaces between the fronds or villi of the placenta (from which the baby obtained by selective absorption all the substances necessary for its development) is forced back into the veins and spongy lining layer of the uterus, making them tense and congested. These are kept under pressure by the muscle layer of the uterus, which, having retracted, does not allow the blood from these tense veins to drain back into the maternal blood stream. During this process, the cord is still pulsating, and some of the foetal blood residual in the placenta is 'pumped' back into the baby, thus allowing further thickening of the placental wall.[46, 47]

When the uterus contracts again (and there is evidence that contractions are stronger at the placental site than elsewhere in the third stage)[48] the congested veins burst and the small amount of extravasated blood causes tearing of the very fine septa of the spongy layer, thereby detaching it from its uterine site. With the same contractions, the criss-crossed muscle fibres surrounding the maternal blood vessels seal off the torn end as the placenta is detached (these fibres are referred to by many as 'living ligatures'). Because of the simultaneous sealing of the blood vessels and the peeling off of the placenta, the blood lost is only in the order of 60–100 ml (2–3 fl oz). The placenta normally separates from the centre, and then descends into the cavity of the uterus, pushed in the direction of least resistance which is the lower portion of the uterus and the cervix, peeling off the membranes as it does so. This process is usually so rapid that contraction and retraction of the cervix do not take place before the placenta is expelled without resistance into the vagina. If the mother is sitting on her haunches, it will fall out of the vagina by gravity,[43] and the small quantity of blood lost in this case (see above) will be kept inside the inverted sac of placenta and membranes. If separation is not quite symmetrical, the placenta will slide down sideways, and the blood escapes from the vagina. Following the expulsion of the placenta the uterus can reduce in size still further, the contraction and retraction of the muscles ensuring that the 'living ligatures' are tightened further.

This process relies on the ability of the uterus to contract and retract rapidly throughout, and initially to contract against a compressed, compact placenta. Any interference may jeopardize the mother's safety by increasing the time before which the living ligatures can act effectively. If the cord is clamped, a counter-resistance is set up in the placenta, the extra foetal blood being trapped within it, and it cannot become compressed and compact. Retraction of the uterus may then be prevented and separation slowed, with consequent delay in the sealing off of the torn blood vessels.

If the placenta cannot separate by rapidly peeling off (like a postage stamp from a rapidly inflated balloon), it will try to separate by the formation of a large blood clot behind the placenta, which is formed from the oozing of the torn but incompletely sealed blood vessels. This is not normal, but abnormal.[43] By the time the placenta has separated by this method, not only has more blood been lost from the mother's circulation to form the clot, but the cervical muscle has also retracted and this combined with a more bulky placenta will make expulsion of the placenta more difficult, if not impossible. The longer the placenta remains undelivered, the greater is the likelihood of more bleeding, as the uterus cannot contract down firmly whilst the bulky placenta is still inside it. This state of affairs is compounded if the uterus is handled at this time, as 'fundal fiddling' may detach the membranes at one point, allowing the retroplacental blood to escape without clotting, thereby further increasing the blood loss and further delaying the complete separation of the placenta.[47] The increased incidence of retained placenta, necessitating a general anaesthetic and manual removal, is itself associated with an increase in blood loss.[43]

In 1978 Walsh[49] and Botha[43] conducted studies in which a group of mothers who received no routine oxytocics prior to placental delivery and had had cord clamping delayed was compared with a control group who had no routine oxytocics but had the cord clamped immediately. Walsh found that the duration of the third stage was the same in both groups (about ten minutes), but that the blood loss after delivery of the placenta was doubled in the early-clamped group (133 ml as against 67 ml) and the total blood loss in the early-clamped group was also significantly higher than the late-clamped group (364 ml as against 268 ml). Moreover, there were retained placenta requiring manual removal in 9 per cent of the cases in the early-clamped group, and *none* in the late-clamped group. In all cases the retention was due to faulty separation and not to faulty implantation.

Botha found that the mean duration of the third stage was far less when the cord was not clamped (4 minutes *v.* 12 minutes) and that the total blood loss was also far less in the unclamped group – an approximate range of 16 ml to 182 ml compared with 100 to 371 ml. Among the mothers in the late-clamped group were two who had postpartum haemorrhages in previous deliveries, and who lost only 450 ml (15 fl oz) and 120 ml (4 fl oz) respectively in the trial. By contrast, the early-clamped group had one mother who lost 780 ml (26 fl oz) and required intervention to prevent further bleeding.

It is interesting to note that the total blood loss in the Walsh study was greater than that of the Botha study, despite the fact that the cords were unclamped in both studies, and it is possible that this may reflect the method of placental delivery – in the Walsh study the placenta was delivered by fundal pressure on a contracted uterus, and in the Botha study the placenta 'was not handled until the mother felt the urge to bear down herself, and was only received when it appeared outside the vagina'.[43] It has been argued that 'compressing or pushing the uterus downwards towards the pelvic cavity . . . contuses and bruises the uterine wall and causes a passive congestion of the uterus which may produce bleeding during subsequent relaxation'.[47]

A further maternal hazard associated with cord clamping is that of isoimmunization (that is, stimulating the production of antibodies in the mother by allowing foetal blood cells to escape into her blood stream). As the placenta separates (physiologically), some foetal blood from the placenta escapes into the torn blood vessels of the maternal circulation. This appears to happen to a varying degree in all pregnancies[50] but it is the rhesus-negative mother carrying the rhesus-positive baby who may be affected by the 'transfusion', if it is great enough to stimulate antibody production. (*Small* transfusions do not appear to provoke antibody production.) It has been postulated that as much as 215 ml of foetal blood may be trapped in the placenta by early clamping of the cord, with a subsequent rise in pressure within this closed system, and that when the uterus contracts (particularly following the use of an oxytocic agent in the third stage) the further increase in pressure – as much as 150 mmHg – has been sufficient to burst the tensely distended umbilical vessels. It is suggested that such circumstances might facilitate the passage of foetal cells into the maternal circulation.[51] This suggestion is supported by work done in the mid-sixties by Doolittle and

Moritz,[52] by Berriman in 1970 and more recently by Ladipo, who found the incidence of foeto–maternal transfusion was doubled when the cord was clamped, compared with no clamping – 66 per cent *v.* 33 per cent.[50] Weinstein *et al.*[53] confirmed the suggestion that oxytocic drugs given before placental delivery also increased the incidence of foeto–maternal transfusion.

Since the introduction of anti-D immunoglobulin (to be administered to rhesus–negative mothers within 36 hours of delivery of a rhesus-positive baby), the incidence of rhesus-negative mothers developing antibodies after the birth of their first child has been dramatically reduced,[54] but failures still occur if the foeto–maternal transfusion is large[50] and any procedure which will reduce the magnitude and incidence of third-stage transfusions (i.e. late clamping of the cord, and not giving oxytocics prior to placental delivery) will reduce the number of mothers thus affected.

Considered purely from the maternal point of view, it would appear from the evidence discussed that the treatment of choice in cases of low risk would be to allow a physiological third stage (i.e. no oxytocic drugs prior to delivery of the placenta, and leaving the cord unclamped or cutting it and allowing it to bleed freely), and in cases of high risk, to give oxytocin prior to delivery of the placenta, treating the cord in the same manner as for low-risk cases, and backing up the oxytocin by the use of ergometrine in selected cases.[55]

Leaving the cord unclamped, or cutting it and allowing free bleeding, obviate the problems of transplacental haemorrhage and interference with the separation of the placenta, and therefore of increased blood loss; but the situation is 'complicated' by the fact that the baby is on the other end of the cord. . . . The only physiological sequence of events for the baby is that described at the beginning of this section: if the cord *is* cut or clamped before the placenta is delivered, the baby may receive less than his physiological 'quota' of blood, and if oxytocin is given prior to placental delivery, the baby may receive more than his quota if the cord *is not* clamped or cut.

Montgomery[56] considered the treatment of the umbilical cord in some detail, with reference particularly to the welfare of the baby. During any mammalian birth, the expulsion of the placenta follows a short time after that of the baby. In the intervening period, the young newly-born is either at its mother's feet if she is standing, or near her vulva if she is lying down, and unless the cord is torn during expulsion or chewed off by the mother, it remains intact until the placenta is delivered. When ultimately severed, the cord is not tied or clamped in any way. 'This mechanism, which evidently evolved for a purpose, provides the newborn with its full allotment of blood from the placenta and assures that no stagnant blood is then retained within the stump of the umbilical cord.' He also points out that the only difference between general mammalian and early human reproduction was that the cord was severed in the case of the human by rubbing it between two stones rather than by chewing it in half. (Whatever method is used, the umbilical stump shrivels and drops off in three to ten days, and the neat navel or 'tummy button' is left, the shape of which is determined by nature, not man!) Tying of the cord was never employed until the ligature became common practice in surgery.

As the physician became more skilful with the use of haemostats [clamps], scissors and ligatures, the umbilical cord presented an inviting site for surgical procedure, and the present custom of immediate severance and immediate ligation of the cord followed. Ligation of the cord makes it possible to get babies and mothers out of the delivery room more rapidly, just as low forceps contribute to more rapid care. Whether they have added to the ultimate welfare of the newborn is a question.[56]

Various workers have shown that vital physiological changes take place in the heart and lungs of the baby in the moments following birth. It has been suggested that the uninterrupted flow of blood through the cord vessels from the 'reservoir' of placental blood acts as a safety valve and 'volume-maintenance system' as adjustments in circulation take place in the heart and circulatory system of the baby.

The flow of blood from placenta to baby is under the influence of gravity, uterine contractions and the onset of respiration in the newborn, and Montgomery maintains that immediate clamping of the cord interferes with the physiological chain of events, in particular the return to the foetal circulation of 75–125 ml ($2\frac{1}{2}$–4 fl öz) of blood, and it also traps in the cord 'stagnant blood which provides an inviting culture medium for bacterial growth'. He advocated delaying the clamping and division of the cord until fifteen to twenty minutes after the delivery of the placenta. Apart from condemning the administration of oxytocic drugs in the third stage (discussed in the previous section), Montgomery also criticizes the practice of cord stripping (or 'milking' the blood from the cord by pinching it between finger and thumb and stroking it towards the baby). He says that this procedure 'brings at each stroke some 10–15 cc of blood quite abruptly into the foetal circulation. It is the equivalent almost of introducing within 1–2 seconds 200 ml of blood into the adult circulation (which could cause heart failure) [author's parenthesis]. It is difficult to understand how the delicate circulatory channel of the newborn can accommodate this blood so abruptly.' Moss *et al.*[57] have suggested that the only time it might be of value as a procedure is following Caesarean section, when it might compensate for the absent uterine contractions and possibly reduce chilling of the baby which might occur while waiting for the cord to cease pulsating. But they too admit that the problem is knowing precisely how much and how long the cord should be stripped.

On the basis of information currently available, Moss *et al.* in their review article felt it reasonable to assume that delayed clamping of the umbilical cord is associated with an increase in blood volume.[57] Yao and Lind[58] estimated that the total blood volume of a newborn baby varied between 65 ml/kg (if the cord was clamped at birth) to 120 ml/kg (if the cord was clamped at three minutes). Assuming an average birth weight of $7\frac{1}{2}$ lb (3.38 kg), this means a range of 219–405 ml of blood. This confirms earlier work by Oh, Oh and Lind in which they found that 'when the cord clamping was delayed by five

minutes the blood volume increased by 61 per cent to 126 ml/
kg'. Again assuming an infant of 7½ lb, the range is 263 (per
100 per cent) to 425 ml.[59] This is consistent with the statement
made in a letter to the *British Medical Journal* (28 July 1973,
p. 236) derived from Davies (*Foetal and Neonatal Physiology*,
Chicago Year Book Medical Publishers, 1968) that 'it is estimated that (particularly if ergometrine is given to the mother
and the cord not clamped) a baby can receive a volume of
blood from the placenta equivalent to as much as half its
entire blood volume after delivery'. It is possible that this may
be more than was intended physiologically. Vardi[60] investigated the extra blood transfused by gravity and delaying cord
clamping, and concluded that the baby received an extra 89
ml of blood. Williams[61] writing in 1909, well before the routine use of third-stage oxytocic drugs, refers to Budin, who
showed that if the cord is not tied early, the baby may received
an extra 92 ml of blood.

If it is the case that the extra blood that 'should' be transfused physiologically is approximately equal to 100 ml rather
than the 200 ml which are apparently received if oxytocics are
given, it would explain the observations of J. M. Gate and
colleagues[62] that the baby is overtransfused as a result of the
'almost universal use of oxytocics to expedite placental separation'. He says that in these circumstances the placenta is
squeezed like a sponge and the baby may receive a blood
transfusion it does not need. 'One would expect the surplus
blood to be haemolysed and that could well be the source of
the bilirubin [the pigment giving rise to yellowing of the skin
when in excess – 'jaundice'] which is causing anxiety to our
paediatric colleagues.'

It would also explain the findings of Yao and Lind[63] that
the large placental transfusion which the baby receives if cord
clamping is delayed has been observed by them to distend
acutely the circulatory system of the normal newborn, who,
despite possessing 'a great capability to adapt to this circulatory overloading, show evidence of increased effort and duration in the extrauterine adaptive processes'. They say,
however, that no harmful effects have been shown to follow

as a result in normal full-term babies. (They do not say whether or not the mothers of the babies thus observed received oxytocic drugs prior to placental delivery.)

On the other side of the coin, it has been suggested that idiopathic respiratory distress (IRDS) may be a consequence of clamping the cord too early. In this case the baby is deprived of his full complement of placental blood and the increased volume of blood required by the pulmonary circulation must be drawn from the baby's own blood stream.[64] Dr Courtney, writing in the *British Medical Journal*, remarks, 'Hypovolaemia [low blood volume] seems a logical cause for failure of pulmonary [lung] expansion which this simple precaution [delaying cord clamping] helps to prevent. . . . If the cord is pulsating well it is important not to cut it [the baby] off from this significant, warm, oxygenated blood transfusion.'[65]

He felt that this extra blood was even more significant in preventing IRDS if the baby was premature or small for dates, an opinion borne out by the work of Moss, Duffie and Fagan, whose study found an increased incidence of IRDS in premature babies whose cords were clamped before the onset of respiration.[66] Most research on the subject has been carried out on normal full-term infants and the exact relationship, if any, of cord clamping to IRDS remains the subject of considerable controversy.[57]

Moss *et al.* in their review article conclude:

In full-term, vigorous infants, 'early' versus 'late' clamping is not a vital issue [in physiological terms]. These babies seem to endure the physiologic consequences of either . . . with no apparent untoward effects. In depressed full-term infants (those slow to breathe or respond) the factor of time may be more significant, since further insult may not be so well tolerated. In premature infants, even if not depressed, the issue assumes still greater importance.

Circumstances alter cases, and nowhere does this happen so rapidly as in the practice of obstetrics and perinatology. It may not be possible to attend satisfactorily to mother or baby with the cord still intact if either need swift medical attention:

neither is it possible to deliver a baby with the cord wrapped tightly round its neck without clamping, cutting and unwinding it. . . . But where the labour and delivery are normal in all respects, and particularly if no oxytocic drugs are given prior to delivery, it would appear to be detrimental to mother and baby to clamp the cord before the placenta is delivered.

The issue of early versus late cord clamping remains a controversial issue for the medical profession (if not for mothers), and further investigations are needed if the issue is to be decided scientifically. Until then, the final word may be left to Laing who, at the International Society for Psychosomatic Obstetrics and Gynaecology meeting in 1972, said, 'And I should like to know why in our society the cord might not be left to be cut as late as possible, rather than as quickly as possible.'[67]

Methods of placental delivery

Whilst it is the case that a good proportion of mothers are concerned about the way in which the umbilical cord is managed in the interest of their babies, and a few may have strong feelings about the routine use of syntometrine, relatively few will have considered the way in which their placenta will be delivered, or the implications of the method chosen by the labour attendant (the doctor or midwife). In Western societies, placental delivery methods are described as either 'maternal effort' (the so-called 'natural' method), or 'mechanical', involving some form of pushing, pulling or uterine manipulation.

As has been seen in the previous section, physiological placental separation occurs when the uterus contracts strongly and the placenta, made thick and compact by the 'escape' of foetal blood via the intact cord to the baby, peels off the uterus at the 'perforation layer'. The placenta then folds in on itself and is pushed towards the lower portion of the uterus by the strongly contracting upper portion or fundus. This process happens so quickly that no retraction has yet taken place in the cervix, and the placenta is 'expelled without resistance into the vagina' . . . after which it will 'fall out by gravity'.[68] This presupposes that a physiological position is adopted for the third stage, so that gravity can act in the same plane as the vagina. Botha recounts that attending 26,000 Bantu mothers over a ten-year period, he rarely had to deal with a retained placenta (and if he did, it normally entailed only lifting out the terminal part of the membranes from the vagina), and never had to resort to blood transfusion for a postpartum haemorrhage.

An undrugged, cooperative mother in a Western hospital may if permitted push out her own placenta unaided. But she will have to do so when the midwife urges rather than when her own inclinations prompt her (unless the two happily co-incide), as she will very probably have been given an oxytocic drug (i.e. syntometrine) with the birth of the baby's first shoulder. As has been mentioned in the section discussing oxytocic drugs, the ergometrine component will come into operation within seven minutes of intramuscular administration, and the placenta needs to be delivered before this happens, lest it be trapped behind the closed, contracted cervix.

The other problem faced by the mother is likely to be the position in which she finds herself: she is very likely to be lying flat, and the sensations of the uterus as it contracts once the baby is born are quite unlike the powerful, positive 'bearing-down' sensations of the second stage. No stage of labour can accurately or aptly be likened to the act of defaecation, which has connotations of 'getting rid of waste material', and also serves to confuse a mother whose baby in the second stage is travelling in quite the opposite direction: but one may wonder how many of those who urge a mother to expel her placenta when lying flat have ever tried to evacuate their bowels in a similar position? Certainly, it will require more effort from her than from her 'primitive' counterpart.

Pulling on the cord to effect delivery of the placenta probably became fashionable in the West following the translation into English of Mauriceau's treatise (1673). He recommended this procedure as he feared that the uterus might close before the placenta was delivered spontaneously.[68] For the next hundred years it was the 'recognized procedure of experienced accoucheurs'.[69] However, any interference with the normal physiological process of parturition, as has been illustrated throughout this book, is accompanied by disadvantages as well as its intended advantages. In the case of cord traction, these are: (a) pulling off or snapping a cord, either because it is very delicate or inserted into the membranes rather than the substance of the placenta; (b) pulling out a placenta which had not completely separated from the lining of the uterus, and consequently leaving a portion behind; and (c) inverting the uterus by pulling on the cord when the placenta is still completely attached.

Pulling off the cord is not in itself detrimental to the mother. If she can deliver the placenta herself by maternal effort, all is well. If it is delivered by other mechanical means, i.e. pushing on the uterus, there are all the disadvantages associated with that technique; if a manual removal is required either because syntometrine has taken full effect and the cervix is closed, and therefore the placenta cannot be delivered by other means, the situation is more serious. Patterson[70] in addition to the above, recalls the need for a flying squad to attend a 'shocked patient without much blood loss but with the placenta in utero and the cord avulsed'. Leaving a portion of the placenta behind is a serious matter as severe bleeding may result if the uterus is unable to contract properly and manual removal is necessary. If the retained fragments are not noticed at the time of delivery, they may become infected and/or give rise to secondary bleeding, which will then require antibiotics, manual removal and possibly a blood transfusion. It may even result in a generalized blood stream infection (septicaemia) and other complications.[70]

Inversion of the uterus (which may be complete and in which the fundus of the uterus is visible between the mother's thighs, or partial, in which case the fundus is not externalized) will result in a state of profound maternal shock and possibly haemorrhage.[71]

Although Crede in 1853 agreed that in the hands of accomplished obstetricians, cord pulling was a satisfactory method, he showed that complications were frequently encountered by the unskilled.[70] Consequently, he devised a method of manual compression of the uterus at the height of a contraction, expressing the placenta thereby. This method is now considered by most obstetricians to be dangerous, although a few still use it. Dame Josephine Barnes (as she is now) writing in 1955 stated:

Maternal shock may follow an attempt to deliver the placenta by Crede's method. The dangers of forcible manipulation of the uterus cannot be overemphasized and indeed Crede's method has now been entirely abandoned by many obstetricians who feel that they prefer manual removal of the placenta as the safer method.[71]

The other alternative was fundal pressure, pushing downwards on the contracted uterus and using it as a sort of piston or battering ram. This, besides having 'no useful effect if the placenta is still in the uterine cavity, whether separated or not',[72] may cause bruising and contusing of the uterine wall, and a passive congestion of the uterus which may cause bleeding when the uterus relaxes.[69] It may also result in a prolapse of the cervix into the vagina as a result of the strain placed upon the uterine ligaments.[73, 74] (It is also painful!)

Ahlfeld, who worked with Crede, found that the same complications condemned by his teacher in the cord-traction method occurred not infrequently when expression was performed by 'incompetent midwives'.[70] He therefore postulated his famous doctrine of 'Hands off the uterus'. Writing more recently, Patterson stated that 'the oldtimers learnt in a hard school, and through the experience which has been built up by midwives for centuries. They knew that the commonest cause of third-stage trouble was fiddling about. It still is, and it behoves us to remember it.'[75] Cord traction, however, became popular once again with the wider use of oxytocic drugs in the 'active management of the third stage'. The remedy of some obstetricians to the problem of fundal fiddling was 'decisive action'.

From the point of view of training undergraduates and pupil midwives, decisive action is more easily presented and more readily accepted than tentative inaction, with its associated temptations. The popularity of cord traction with the midwifery staff indicates the attractions which the method holds.[76]

In some cases, the attendants would await the classic signs of (separation and) descent – namely, an escape of blood, lengthening of the cord and rising up of the uterus – before attempting to pull on the cord, but others regarded these signs as unreliable and often missed in the general activity of the delivery: they therefore advocated cord traction immediately the uterus had contracted, with the free hand 'guarding' the uterus to prevent uterine inversion (a modification of the technique described by Brandt, who advocated pushing the uterus *upwards* with the free hand). Some go even further, and recommend cutting the cord immediately the baby is delivered and immediately pulling on the cord, with the other hand pressing the uterus upwards and backwards. Continuous traction is applied, so that the instant of placental separation is recognized by a slackening of tension in the cord, which is then delivered by further traction (the 'cord sign of separation'). All this, having first given syntometrine with the delivery of the baby's first shoulder.[77]

If mechanical methods of delivering the placenta, as described above, fail, resort must be made to manual removal. This entails giving the mother a general anaesthetic so that a hand may be passed into the uterus to separate the placenta, with the fingers moving from side to side. This procedure, whilst life-saving in *some* situations, is not without its hazards both in terms of damage to the uterus and anaesthetic complications. The complications of cord traction may be rare, but they do still occur; and in the year in which Fliegner and Hibbard published their paper advocating the 'Active Management of the Third Stage of Labour',[76] there were three cases in the Salisbury General Infirmary alone of acute inversion of the uterus for which active management was responsible.[78] Furthermore 'there seems little doubt that this hazard is increased if an active policy of management of the third stage is practised'.[78]

The development of the techniques and drugs necessary for the pursuance of such a policy has meant that they have been, and undoubtedly will continue to be lifesaving in some circumstances, and dramatically reduce the PPH rate in others. But that is not necessarily an argument for applying them routinely. The situation in which they were shown to reduce the PPH rate most dramatically and significantly was when the third stage lasted for over thirty minutes;[76] but in the majority of cases the normal third stage lasts only about one-third of this time. Botha and Walsh, who managed the third stage physiologically (no oxytocic drugs and no cord clamping) found an average duration of ten minutes and no manual removals required. Third-stage delay was the situation in which Patterson,[70] a staunch opponent of routine active management, himself recommended cord traction 'with early resort to manual removal should cord traction prove ineffective'.

When the mother is not deemed to be at risk, and has had a normal first and second stage, she 'could be allowed to complete the process normally'.[79] One GP obstetrician, formerly a supporter of the active approach to the third stage, confesses to having reversed his opinion and reverted to the old-fashioned management, being now 'utterly convinced of its superiority'. He concludes in his letter to the *BMJ*, 'It is gratifying and instructive to see how well the uterus will do its job if left alone.'[80]

The newborn baby

Gentle birth

Dr Fredrick Leboyer published his book, *Birth without Violence*,[81] in 1975, at a time when many people were expressing their concern at the widespread use of drugs in labour, routine separation of the baby from its mother, and the increase in the use of obstetric techniques – e.g. induction, monitoring and forceps deliveries. The focus of his book (and also his film) was that birth should be a gentle transition from the womb to the outside world, rather than a tidal wave of 'sensation'. To this end he suggested specific actions which he believed would minimize the 'shock' of being born: a dark, quiet room, placing the baby on the mother's abdomen, delaying cord clamping, massaging the baby and placing him in a warm bath.

Although Leboyer was at pains to impress upon those who questioned him that he wished to impart an *attitude* and not a technique, his procedures became the subject of considerable controversy. Delivering in the dark, delaying cord cutting and bathing the baby received particular criticism.[82-84] It is not difficult for even a sympathetic audience to find objections to some of Leboyer's actions and assumptions. There is now some evidence[85] that towards the end of pregnancy the baby is not in total darkness in the uterus, but that enough light can penetrate the mother's stretched abdominal and uterine walls to allow a diffuse pink glow throughout the amniotic fluid, rather like holding one's hand over the end of a torch. The intensity of this glow will depend on the brightness of the external light and the thickness of the clothing covering the abdomen, but it may be reasonable to suggest that the newborn infant has some knowledge and even some 'expectation' of light, so that darkness may be just as strange as overhead fluorescent lights. From the practical point of view, the birth attendant must obviously have enough light to see what he or she is doing, and an immediate source of *bright* light should the situation suddenly warrant it.

There are similar objections to trying to deliver a baby into silence. There is good evidence[86] that the womb is quite a noisy place: there is a very loud, continuous, rhythmical, 'whooshing' sound, which is punctuated by occasional rumbles of air. Researchers have found that the baby also responds to external sound (independent of what his mother hears), but that this had to be very loud indeed to exceed that which the baby is constantly hearing. Silence as the baby is born is not only likely to be strange for the baby, but will also impose considerable restraints on the mother, father and midwife, and 'rob' the baby of the cries of joy and spontaneous greetings that are characteristic of normal undrugged deliveries. Lind,[87] who had 130 normal full-term births photographed, felt that the expressions on the faces of the babies confirmed his impression that a normal delivery is not as a rule a painful experience for a child. In his photographs none of the babies showed signs of anxiety or pain, but rather curiosity and great expectation, despite not being delivered into a silent environment.

Bathing the baby immediately after delivery may indeed cause a drop in its temperature, which is the objection usually put forward by critics of Leboyer's technique, but presumably this could be avoided if the room temperature were high enough. It is, however, quite likely that 'high enough' is considerably higher than anyone else in the room could find comfortable (or economical!) The McMaster study[88] which compared babies delivered at 27 degrees Centigrade and given a warm water bath with babies delivered at 24 degrees and *not* bathed, found that the underarm temperatures of the bathed group were significantly lower than those of the controls for up to one hour following delivery – although none was dangerously low, i.e. below 35 degrees. This suggests, among other things, that room temperature needs to be well above 27 degrees Centigrade (80 degrees Fahrenheit) to avoid cooling the baby. (The alternative would be to use a servo-controlled infra-red heater, positioned about 28 inches above the baby.[89] The McMaster study also found that 'the Leboyer bath did not appear to have a calming effect: of the 19 babies observed, 9 reacted with irritable crying and 10 maintained or achieved an alert state.'

However, the debate over the details of the Leboyer birth cannot detract from the central issue – Leboyer's belief in the baby as an important, sensitive individual who should be treated as gently and respectfully as the situation will allow. It may or may not be possible to prove that his approach confers measurable long-term benefits (Rappoport's uncontrolled follow-up study[90] suggested that development was generally superior in infants delivered by Leboyer's 'method'); but then proof is not generally required to substantiate the assertion that it is better to treat adults gently rather than roughly or thoughtlessly.

The only scientific randomized trial applied to the Leboyer technique to date was conducted at the McMaster University Medical Center.[88] Although it produced some very interesting results, it failed to find any clear-cut differences in either the mother's perception of her birth experience or in the behaviour of the baby, whether during the neonatal period or at eight months of age. The researchers did point out, however, that there were only minimal differences between the two methods of delivery used: 'The control deliveries though more conventional were intended to be equally gentle, and differed from the Leboyer group only in location, lighting, room temperature, draping, time of cord clamping, type of contact with the mother (in both groups the mother held her baby immediately after birth) and bath.' They felt that they could not ethically compare 'the Leboyer protocol with the anachronistic practices which he and many others had condemned', and set up their study 'to avoid confounding the controversial specifics of Leboyer's method with the *principles of gentleness*' (author's emphasis).

It could therefore be argued that their *attitude* to birth and the baby was already similar to that of Leboyer, and that although they pay sufficient attention to the wishes of expectant parents in their hospital to provide Leboyer deliveries for those who request them (which is what prompted the study), it may be that in their institution it is simply 'gilding the lily'.

It is difficult to see, as they point out, how anyone could ethically compare 'Leboyer' practices with 'anachronistic practices' in the same institution/study, and it may be that Leboyer's principles will not be satisfactorily subjected to the scientific application of a randomized controlled trial. If they are accepted, it will be because mothers *want* them and feel them to be 'right'. In the meantime, it is possible to argue against specific practices which are a feature of many conventional deliveries.

The routine extraction of mucus from the baby's nose and mouth

In hospital, nearly all babies are subjected to the routine suctioning of their nose and mouth 'to clear the airway', without any regard to whether or not such a procedure is necessary. The suction is usually performed with a bulb syringe or a nasogastric mucus extractor with a glass trap. Most babies born normally and unaffected by drugs have their nose and mouth cleared spontaneously as they are born by the pressure exerted on the chest wall by the vagina, and breathing begins within seconds of the chest being delivered. To subject a baby who is breathing peacefully to oral and nasal suction 'just in case' is a totally unnecessary assault.

Babies who have difficulty in breathing (and it is five times more common in hospital than at home)[91] are far more likely to owe their problems to the use of narcotics and anaesthetics in labour (and/or the reasons for their use) than to a blocked airway, and if this is the case, mucus extraction will not improve the situation. Dr Donald Garrow, Consultant Paediatrician at Amersham, High Wycombe and Stoke Mandeville hospitals, with special knowledge of cardiac and respiratory rhythms in newborn babies) has said, 'Sticking a catheter down a baby's throat is bad: pushing it into a baby's nose and mouth does nothing at all to help it breathe. Mucus catheters should be banned as dangerous instruments.'[92] Pushing a mucus extractor 'blindly' into the nasopharynx, larynx or trachea of the baby, via the nose or mouth, may stimulate the endings of the vagus nerve which are situated there. If the vagus nerve is stimulated, the impulses will pass over the vagal network to the medulla (the part of the brain which contains the respiratory and cardiac centres). The net result is a disturbance of rhythm, slowing or even stopping of the heart, and inhibition or cessation of breathing (apnoea). In a study conducted at the New Haven Medical Center, researchers found that following 'blind' nasopharyngeal suction, of 46 infants, 7 of them developed serious slowing of the heartbeat; 1 (of these 7) had a cardiac arrest (i.e. the heart stopped beating altogether), and 5 (of the same 7) stopped breathing.

The authors conclude that blind suction of the nasopharynx is a hazardous procedure, particularly in the first critical minutes of life when the baby is physiologically unstable, and they suggest that their results are sufficiently serious 'to warrant re-examination and careful clinical evaluation of the use of the nasopharyngeal catheter immediately after birth'.[93] In instances where thick mucous blood or meconium is thought to be obstructing the baby's lungs, it should be removed under direct vision by a paediatrician. The use of a bulb syringe may be unpleasant and in many cases unnecessary, but the bulb cannot usually reach the larynx or trachea and is therefore less likely to cause damage.

Holding the baby upside down

It is still the practice in a great many hospitals to hold the baby upside down, suspended by the ankles, for the purpose of allowing 'any fluid in the trachea to drain out'[94] and facilitate breathing. While in this position, the baby may also be smacked on the bottom to startle him/her into crying.

These practices show a total disregard for the baby as an independent human being. The newborn baby has been shown repeatedly to be acutely sensitive in his perceptions, and it must be a terrifying sensation to be suddenly hung upside down in space, having just come from the confines of the womb. Dr Leboyer's photograph of a screaming newborn baby with its fists clenched by its face[95] speaks volumes on the subject of the needless suffering imposed upon the newborn. Moreover, this suffering is not solely psychological. Dr Robert Salter (Emeritus Professor of Orthopaedic Surgery at the Toronto Hospital for Sick Children) has condemned this practice (of suspending babies by the feet) because of the enormous strain it places on the hip joints. Such straining may, he says, cause untold damage which may lead to serious complications later on. He further adds that this potential damage may be compounded if the baby has its bottom slapped whilst being held in this position, as this can further damage the hip joints.[96]

There are less traumatic and more effective ways of clearing the air passages should the need arise.

Wrapping the baby up immediately

One of the chief concerns of midwives and doctors, once the baby is born safely and breathing properly, is that he/she shall not cool down. A wet newborn baby cools down very rapidly for several reasons: the room temperature is usually very much lower than that of the amniotic fluid/uterus from which he has just come, his surface area is large in relation to his body weight, and his metabolic response is not sufficient to compensate for his rapid heat loss.[97]

If a newborn baby is allowed to get cold and stay cold, the consequences may be serious. The baby will use up all his available energy stores in trying to keep himself warm, which may lead to hypoglycaemia (low blood sugar).[98] 'Cold stress' may also delay the baby's adjustment from foetal to newborn circulation[99] and adversely affect thyroid, adrenal, water and fat metabolism.[100-102]

For these very good reasons, the usual response of the birth attendants is to dry the infant thoroughly and wrap him in a warm blanket, leaving only a small amount of the face exposed. This is an effective way to cut down heat loss, but it unfortunately has the effect of greatly altering the mother's interaction with her baby in the first minutes after birth. (This is compounded if the baby is removed from the mother's arms and placed in a heated crib. This has been done in the past in the belief that the baby would be warmer in a crib, but a study conducted in 1974[97] suggests that this belief is mistaken. The study, carried out on normal babies (over 5 lb, no breathing problems, high Apgar score, normal delivery) compared the body temperature of babies placed in cribs with those placed in their mothers' arms at five and sixteen minutes after birth. They found that 'the temperatures of both groups remained within the acceptable range of heat loss . . . and . . . the differences in the mean temperatures of the two groups was not significant.')

Klaus and Kennell filmed 12 mothers with their full-term

infants, allowing each mother total freedom in handling her baby, by placing them both under a radiant heater to prevent them from getting cold.[103] They found that each mother went through an 'orderly and predictable' pattern of behaviour when she first examined her infant. She began hesitantly to touch the baby's hands and feet with her finger tips, and within four or five minutes began to caress the baby's body with the palms of her hands. This intense examination continued for several minutes, and then diminished as the mother dozed off with the naked infant at her side.

Macfarlane[104] found that his own observations of mothers' initial contact with their newborn babies in a conventional delivery room 'differed in many ways from Klaus and Kennell's . . . because in this situation the baby was well wrapped up and the only exposed parts were his head and face, and sometimes small, pink hands and feet!' Other researchers comparing the effects of early contact with delayed contact have specifically given the early contact groups their *naked* babies.[105, 106] Not only does placing mother and baby under a radiant heater facilitate this spontaneous 'examination' of the newborn by its mother, but it also appears to be more effective in preventing heat loss than the usual procedure of wrapping. Dahm and James[107] compared five groups of infants: three groups were in room air 22.5–26.5 degrees Centigrade (72.5–79.7 degrees Fahrenheit) with one group wet, one group dry and one group both dry and wrapped, and two groups were under a radiant heater, one wet and one dried. They found that the heat loss in wet infants exposed to room air was five times as great as in those that were both dried and warmed. The temperatures of babies dry and wrapped were similar to those of babies wet and warmed, and none were quite as good as those dried and warmed. They conclude,

In vigorous infants, the simple manoeuvre of drying and wrapping in a warm blanket is almost as effective in diminishing heat loss as placing them under a radiant heater. However, in depressed or immature infants who may be more asphyxiated (short of oxygen) or have reduced energy stores, radiant heat maintains body temperature while allowing access to the patient [i.e. the baby].

They also suggest that the heat loss in the 'dry and warmed' group could be reduced still further if the output of the heater was increased (in their study the power was set at 400 watts and was 28 inches above the baby) and air currents in the delivery room were reduced. Some hospitals now have radiant heaters above the delivery beds to facilitate early mother/infant contact without risk of the baby's cooling down,[108] and there seems to be no reason on physiological grounds why their use should not be extended.

The routine removal of the baby to a nursery after birth

It is the custom in all but a very few hospitals to remove the baby from the mother after she has seen it and possibly held it for a short period. There are various 'reasons' given for this practice if the mother should happen to question it (which very few do – such being the effects of institutions): 'The baby needs to rest after the exertions of being born', 'needs weighing', 'cleaning up' or 'warming up'. Sometimes the mother may even be told that the baby needs a 'period of observation'.

Unless the baby is in need of the care of a paediatrician and intensive-care nurses, there is no need to remove him from his mother. Keeping the baby warm has already been discussed: the baby can quite happily 'wait' to be weighed or cleaned until the mother is ready for this to be done, and then it can be done at her bedside. Researchers have shown repeatedly that the normal baby is especially alert and receptive after birth, ready to interact with his mother; any rest he needs he will take later, and unless he is in need of specialist observation, or the mother has been given narcotic drugs, there is no one who will 'observe' her baby better or more keenly than she. Moreover, all these necessary procedures can be and are carried out perfectly satisfactorily at home when that is the place of delivery. In fact, aside from the wish to escape any unnecessary interference during the labour, the desire not to be separated from the baby was the main reason women gave for wanting their confinement at home, according to Sheila Kitzinger's study.[109] She also points out that every single mother in the study who had already had one baby in hospital wrote to this effect on this subject, often at great length. In the letters written to her, many women expressed a passionate sense of urgency about being able to care for their babies themselves from the first seconds of life, and it is a great indictment of our hospitals that they feel this is possible only in the home environment.

Only in our 'civilized' society is the continuum of the mother–baby relationship so regularly interrupted, and it would appear that in some circumstances we may pay a high price for arbitrarily separating mother and baby. A controlled study carried out in Nashville, Tennessee, on 301 mothers and babies[110] found that there was a significantly higher incidence of child abuse or 'parenting disorders' amongst mothers who were deprived of contact with their babies for twelve hours following delivery, and thereafter permitted contact only for thirty minutes every four hours for the next two days; this compared with those who had their babies rooming in after an initial seven-hour period of separation. (It should be stressed that these babies were all normal, vigorous full-term babies, born spontaneously, and both mother and baby remained healthy throughout their stay in hospital.) This study is one of eleven reviewed by Marshall Klaus at the Rainbow Babies' and Children's Hospital Symposium on Parent/Infant Attachment in Cleveland, Ohio, in November 1977.[111] The other ten studies concentrated on early contact, two compared extra contact in the first three hours, plus extra time over the next three days with controls, and eight compared extra time in just the first two hours with controls. He found that, no matter when increased amounts of contact were added in the first three days after birth, there appears to be improved mothering behaviour.

Much of the behaviour which is involved in parenting is learned rather than instinctive.[112] Nevertheless Dr Klaus believes that increased contact with her infant may somehow set in motion a sequence of innate behaviour so that the mother may recapitulate what was previously normal human maternal behaviour (i.e. nearly continuous feeding and carrying of the baby). The Swedish study[106] by Peter de Chateau found that twenty minutes' extra skin-to-skin contact between mother and baby made the woman having had a first baby behave more as if it were her second (or subsequent) in terms of her handling.

The evidence of the past thirty years tends to argue against a 'critical' period for bonding and attachment in humans (bonding is defined by Brazelton as the initial attraction of a mother to her baby and her desire to form an emotional relationship, and attachment is defined as the long hard process of developing the bond). Mothers and infants in Western hospitals have, by and large, had minimal contact, yet most have managed to form close attachments and most mothers have provided adequate mothering (even if their early separation has meant that they will have had to work harder at it, and that a greater proportion has failed to form a satisfactory relationship than might otherwise have done so).[110]

Since the human infant depends for his survival (to a far greater extent than the young of any other species) on his mother bonding with and attending to him, it would seem unlikely that this life-sustaining relationship would be dependent on a single process. Dr Klaus suggests[113] that an analogy may be drawn between the bonding/attachment process and that which triggers the first breath in the newborn. A lengthy search by respiratory physiologists for the 'key' factor which initiated respiration in the newborn baby revealed that there were *many* factors, each of which played some part and that if one or more factors were absent then the combined effect of those that remained would in most cases be sufficient to cause the infant to take his first breath.

Keeping the mother and baby together from birth onwards is likely to facilitate and enhance the many behavioural, hormonal, physiological and immunological mechanisms which serve to bind them together, and they ought not to be separated without very good reasons. MacFarlane summarizes the situation thus: 'For a non-specific time after birth, there does seem to be a period in the developing relationship between mothers, fathers and babies when separation may be detrimental.'[114]

How detrimental the separation is seems to depend on the mother's social class – the better the social environment, the greater is the chance of repairing any damage done at birth. The poorer the social-class environment, the more likely it is that any harm done at birth will be compounded. The impact which social class may have in the longer term on the mother-infant relationship when the two have been separated at birth is illustrated by two separate studies. Leiderman and Seashore[115] studied the effects of separation on three groups of white, middle-class mothers, including two groups whose premature babies had been in a special-care unit for three weeks or more. One group could see but not touch their babies, the second group could touch and handle their babies in the incubators and cots, and the third group had normal-term babies and were not separated.

They found that the separation had little effect on interaction between mothers and babies, although the separated group smiled at and cuddled their babies significantly less than the others in the initial period. At one year, these differences had almost disappeared. The only striking difference found at the twenty-one-month follow-up was that five mothers (out of twenty-two) in the 'no-contact' group had got divorced, one mother in the premature plus contact group was divorced, whilst there were no divorces in the control group.

The study done by Klaus and Kennell,[116] on the other hand, shows striking differences in the attachment behaviour of the mothers and babies in the two groups. The effects of separation were studied in two groups each of fourteen black, inner-city, mostly unmarried mothers of poor social class, none of whom were breast-feeding, all of whom had normal, full-term deliveries. The fourteen control-group mothers were given the traditional American contact with their babies – a glimpse of the baby at birth, a brief visit six to twelve hours later for identification and feeding, and thereafter four-hourly visits of twenty to thirty minutes for feeds. The other group were given their naked babies for one hour within the first three hours after birth, and an extra five hours' contact each afternoon for the next three days – a total of sixteen hours extra contact. Follow-up observations showed that the extra-contact mothers were more likely to pick up and comfort their babies when they cried (even when the mothers knew they were not wet or hungry), stood closer to and were more likely to soothe their babies during physical examinations, and more likely to fondle and hold their babies *en face* during feeding periods. These differences were still obvious at one year, and at two years the children of the extra-contact group of mothers had much better linguistic ability – their mothers used twice as many questions, fewer words per proposition, more adjectives and fewer commands than the control group.

In other words, early separation combined with poor social class may make a substantial difference to maternal behaviour and these effects may continue to manifest themselves for up to two years after delivery.

Chemical separation

If the mother has received drugs during labour (particularly pethidine), the chances of her being able to interact satisfactorily with her baby at birth are reduced. If the drugs are mistakenly given right at the end of labour (a mistake which is more likely to occur if the mother is not examined vaginally prior to the administration of the drug), she may be interested only in going to sleep after the birth, as the sedative aspect of the drug takes effect. If the drug is given earlier in labour, it is the baby who is more likely to be drowsy and unresponsive to his mother's attentions. Unfortunately, this state of affairs in the baby persists possibly for several days, and may interfere with the mother's ability to bond to her infant. It is very difficult to like a person who does not respond to any of your advances, and turns a feeding session into a chore because of the number of times he has to be jostled and coaxed to feed.

It would seem that there is plenty of evidence to support the contention that mothers and babies should not be separated in any way or at any point from birth onwards without good reason, and that when it is essential (e.g. if the baby is premature or requires urgent medical attention) strenuous attempts should be made to give the mother as much physical and emotional access to her baby as is possible.

The effects of hospitalization on the mother–infant relationship

Although many hospitals now have a policy of rooming in, that is, four- to six-bedded wards with the babies beside the mothers' beds during the day, rather than central, American-style nurseries, it is still very common for the baby to be removed from its mother at night, so that it can be observed by the hospital staff. This is particularly true of the first night in hospital, when the mother is assumed to need sleep and is thus given sleeping tablets and the baby is removed.

The mother's need for sleep on the first night following delivery will depend on what time her baby was born. Babies born normally, well and undrugged, commonly feed two or three times in the first hour or so, when they are 'quietly alert' and will then sleep for seven or eight hours if undisturbed. During this time the mother can also sleep if she needs to. However, she also needs to use some of that rest time to begin to come to terms with the birth of the baby, particularly if it is her first, and to relive the events of the labour and delivery in her mind, coupled with frequent glances at the baby by her side to remind herself of his reality. When a baby is born at home, this natural sequence of events can take place uninterrupted and the mother can slowly absorb the vastness and complexity of motherhood and begin to know and care for her baby.

It is very difficult for this to happen in hospital. She cannot mentally order the events of the birth if her mind is clouded with drugs. It is hard enough for her to absorb the fact that she and her husband are now a family, when her husband must go home and leave her; if the baby is removed also it must be almost impossible. If she does not sleep, she may lie awake, emotionally isolated, imagining that every cry she hears is her baby.

Furthermore, a baby whose mother intends to breast-feed him needs to be given the breast when he cries, not water, dextrose or worse still, artificial milk. It will take longer for the mother to build up her milk supply and cause her more discomfort if she misses feeds because her baby is given water or other fluids at night. What is more, a totally breast-fed baby does not need extra water – his fluid and feed intake are perfectly balanced in breast milk. This is true even if the baby is jaundiced: a trial done at Queen Charlotte's Hospital showed that water supplements made no difference to the onset of jaundice, to the mean age of the peak serum bilirubin (bilirubin is the pigment in the blood which causes the 'jaundice' colour) or to the number of babies requiring photo-therapy (treatment under lights).[117] Water is inadequate for the baby if he is hungry, and it cannot be presumed that he is *not* hungry when crying simply because it is less than two hours since his last feed. Many babies who are 'allowed' to feed as often as they want take very variable numbers of feeds during a twenty-four-hour period, with variable intervals. 'In the early days some babies may want feeding every hour or so, and the greatest number of feeds often occurs on the fifth day. In the Sheffield survey . . . 29 per cent of babies wanted eight feeds on the fifth day and 10 per cent wanted more than nine.'[118] Allowing mothers to believe that feeding every three to four hours is the 'norm' for breast-fed babies will only serve to undermine their confidence in their ability to feed their babies properly, just on their own milk, when they find that their baby wants to be fed more frequently.

Other common fallacies perpetuated by many hospitals/ professionals include the notion that it is necessary to 'time' feeds and limit sucking time to two, five and seven and finally to ten minutes in order to prevent sore nipples.[81] Nipple soreness is due to a baby's being incorrectly positioned at the breast. (A baby properly latched on to the breast has the nipple so far back in his mouth that he compresses the milk ducts, which are located well behind the nipple under the areola, between his tongue and the roof of his mouth when he feeds. At no time is he sucking the nipple itself.) The converse of the notion is also true – i.e. it does not matter how short the mother makes the feed – if the baby is not properly latched on, she will get some nipple soreness. Breast-feeding is *not* painful in itself, but it may well become so through incorrect positioning.[119] Mothers may also be told that they should feed the baby from both sides at each feed: if the baby is content and/or asleep after an unrestricted feed at the first breast, then there is nothing else the mother needs to do except remember to offer the other side first next time he wants feeding.

There are other respects (apart from this regular separation of mother and baby and potential impairment of the feeding relationship) in which many hospitals are not good places in which to learn about mothering in the psychological sense. The mother may have no privacy in which to develop a relationship with her baby: single rooms are hard to come by and drawn curtains are rarely respected by professionals, housekeepers or cleaning staff. The mother may be told she must not cuddle her baby (unless he is being fed) for fear of 'spoiling' him: she must not place him or change him on her bed for fear of contaminating him/her – let alone have him actually in her bed – and some hospitals have such a poor opinion of new mothers that they forbid them to carry their newborn babies (despite the fact that in many cases they will be carried for a substantial part of every day once they are home) lest they drop them.

The mother is even encouraged frequently though implicitly to be dependent on the hospital 'experts' in the care of her baby, and not to think for herself. Some even feel it necessary to *ask* if they may change their babies if they wish to do this outside of the scheduled time!

Consequently, many mothers go home with tiny, total strangers whom they may find it very hard even to like, and with no confidence in their own abilities. The time in hospital may be regarded retrospectively as a sort of 'limbo' state and it may be weeks or even months before they can recover their lost self-esteem.

Recommended reading for breastfeeding mothers

David Harvey (ed.), *New Life*, Marshall Cavendish, 1979.
Jenny Stables, *A Mother's Guide to Breastfeeding*, W. H. Allen
& Co. Ltd, 1981
P. and A. Stanway, *Breast is Best*, Pan, 1978

Chapter 8

Alternatives and improvements

Midwifery in Holland

Midwives have been officially sanctioned in Holland since the beginning of the thirteenth century, when they first began working from Catholic convents. The midwife is a member of the medical profession, and like the doctor, her sphere of work is defined by the laws of medicine written in 1856. The first midwifery schools were started in 1865, and now provide a three-year training. A woman who wishes to train as a midwife is not required to be a nurse first, and consequently, there are very few nurses in midwifery in Holland, unlike the situation in Britain where the vast majority of midwives are also nurses.

Once qualified, a midwife is an independent practitioner with professional status, the traditional, national caretaker of the normal birth. Domiciliary (or as they have been known in Britain since 1974, community) midwives work from home and have their own consulting rooms where mothers attend for antenatal care. All mothers are seen once by a physician for a complete physical checkup, but other than this the midwife is responsible for the mother's total care, and is able to form and maintain a one-to-one relationship with the mother throughout the antenatal, natal and postnatal period. If the midwife observes any abnormality, she refers the mother directly to a specialist obstetrician who will then if necessary take over her care.

Iron tablets are not prescribed routinely for pregnant women in Holland, and it is the responsibility of the midwife to check the iron content of the mother's blood and prescribe iron supplements if appropriate.

Since 1925 there has been a special training programme for maternity aid nurses (*Kraamverzorgsten*). These are girls of at least eighteen years of age with a good education who then receive four months' residential instruction and twelve months' practical training in homes. They must also pass an examination, and at the end of their training are adjudged to be competent to 'replace' the mother in the running of the household – housekeeping, shopping, cooking, cleaning, looking after other children, and providing the whole family with an evening meal. In addition, they take over the nursing tasks involved in the postnatal care of mother and baby and help to establish breast feeding. They begin work at seven a.m. and remain in the house until the husband returns in the evening. They work ten consecutive days. The nurses work from a centre with which the mothers will register in early pregnancy (mothers with existing children are given priority).

The Dutch national health insurance scheme pays the midwife's fee and most of the cost of the maternity aid nurse. It will not, however, cover payment for a *planned normal* delivery which takes place in hospital: it is the mother who must pay. In 1974 the average midwife received the equivalent of £55.60 per mother, this including all the antenatal care and delivery as well as eight daily postnatal visits. Since the average midwife can conduct 200 home confinements per year, this meant an average annual income of £11,000, and up to £19,000 for 350 deliveries. (The midwife would of course pay all her own expenses, including the buying of equipment.) The maternity aid nurse in 1974 received £22 per day – an average annual income of £2500–£3000. The general practitioner is not paid to attend unless there is no midwife covering the area, thus affording a degree of financial protection to the midwife. The mother may choose her midwife, doctor, and/or obstetrician, and she may also choose to give birth in a maternity centre or clinic as an alternative to home or hospital.

In 1958, 74 per cent of all Dutch births were at home. By 1975, this figure had dropped to 47 per cent[1] and some midwives are expressing concern about the modern trends in birth in Holland.[2] Foetal monitors, for example, are being used more and more in the hospitals and more women are choosing hospital deliveries with their associated services of epidurals. Also, many women having normal deliveries in hospital are being delivered by doctors. To set up practice as a midwife outside a hospital is becoming more and more difficult. It entails not only a huge financial commitment, but the older established midwives are likely to compete more successfully than newly established ones for the falling numbers of women seeking home deliveries. Consequently, many more midwives are looking for work in a hospital setting.

Midwifery in Denmark

Midwives in Denmark, as in Holland, have centuries of legal tradition behind them, and have high professional status on a par with medicine, the ministry, teaching and the law. Denmark is a small country and has only about five hundred midwives, all of whom train at the Rigshospital in Copenhagen. This national school for midwives produces thirty-three midwives per year. The minimum age for entry to the school is twenty years, but the waiting list is long, and it usually takes several years to gain admittance. The training takes three years (as in Holland) and is paid for mostly by the student, with a small state grant. Again, there is no necessity for the midwifery student to have trained previously as a nurse, and in fact the school prefers not to take nurses for midwifery training, as the two professions are regarded as quite separate. The student midwives spend the entire first year dealing only with normal births, so that they are thoroughly conversant with the normal variations before they see the abnormal. (This is quite different from the British training, where student midwives spend the first part of their training in hospitals where the majority of labours they witness may be heavily 'influenced' by obstetric technology.)

Traditionally, there have been three kinds of midwife in Denmark: the district midwife, assigned to a practice by the local authorities, and relocated according to the needs of different districts; hospital midwives, working alongside physicians within the hospital structure; and independent midwives who book their own clients and were paid by the Danish national health insurance. But as in Holland and Britain at the beginning of the seventies, hospital births have become more fashionable – a form of social status – and furthermore doctors are encouraging women to deliver in hospital. As the number of home births dropped, the independent midwives turned to the government, who responded with a law requiring that every midwife be registered with a hospital, clinic or district. As a result, the independent midwife was assured of a continuing job and income, but sacrificed her independence and can no longer seek her own clients.[3] She may still function in clinics which are separate from the hospital, but must send her high-risk mothers to see a hospital doctor three times during pregnancy. High-risk mothers who are cared for by the hospital doctors are referred to the midwife at least once during the pregnancy.[4] In the case of low-risk mothers, there is total continuity of care antenatally, though a different midwife may do the delivery. Curiously, the midwives do not provide postnatal care, and their interest in the mother and baby following delivery is confined to a visit on the fourth day by the midwife who provided antenatal care, and on the seventh day by the midwife who delivered the mother – in both cases to ask for comments and criticisms of her labour and antenatal care with a view to possible improvements.

Midwifery in Britain

Midwifery in Britain took much longer to receive the official sanction of government, and it was not until 1902 that the

first Midwives Act was passed and state registration of midwives became compulsory by law. The Central Midwives
Board was set up to regulate the training (of three months)
and the practice of midwives, once qualified. The length of
training has gradually been lengthened and from 1938 it was
one year for trained nurses and two years for women with no
previous medical or nursing experience. This training period
has now been increased to eighteen months for qualified
nurses and three years for direct entrants in response to the
'strong representation' made to the House of Commons Social
Services Committee by both the Central Midwives Board and
the Royal College of Midwives to bring Britain into line with
the European Community.[5] (Eighteen months is the minimum
training period compatible with EEC regulations.) The training takes place in one of the 176 training schools throughout
the country and is now 'integrated'; the old system of Part I
and Part II (each of six months and undertaken separately)
has been discontinued. Of pupil midwives 99 per cent are
currently state registered nurses and midwifery training is still
seen by many as a postgraduate qualification, to be obtained
in order to be able to move on or 'up'. CMB reports issued
annually show that only about 50 per cent of midwives practise
at all after qualifying, and that this number is further reduced
in the succeeding years.[6]

There are very few midwifery schools which offer the
three-year training for women who choose to be primarily
midwives, as is the case in Holland and Denmark. Being a
nurse first (a process in which it takes three years to achieve
registration) and a midwife second tends in many cases to
have a profound if insidious effect on the attitude of the
midwife compared with that of her direct entry counterpart.
Student nurses have instilled into them all through their training that they should obey without question the instructions
of those in authority, which ultimately means those of the
doctor: they are working constantly in an atmosphere of pathology, where patients usually enter the hospital to be cured.
Nurses are trained to be watchful of their patients' condition,
ever on the lookout for complications, which are of course

reported to the doctor. Nurses are not often asked for their opinion in the management of a patient's treatment. This is not a good basis on which to enter midwifery, particularly when in many cases the first three months of training, which are spent in hospital, are likely to be spent in an atmosphere of obstetric technology and 'active management' of labour. By the time she begins her community experience the future midwife may well have come to accept that in midwifery, as in nursing, she must be on the lookout for pathology, to the point where she expects that with each labour something will go wrong and require the expert intervention of the obstetrician – and indeed may be mildly surprised when 'occasionally' it does not. Some midwives are able to shake off the legacy of their nursing training and become what Professor Kloosterman calls 'real midwives' but others remain nurse–midwives, that is, nurses first.

We have nurse–midwives in our department. We have midwives and we have nurses. I think the difference is one of character. Our nurse–midwives are split into two kinds of women, the real nurses and the real midwives. There are people who prefer to share responsibility with the doctor and who are very keen on seeing that everything the doctor asks for is done punctually. Of course, we like to work with these nurses. And midwives like to be independent, to give their own opinions. Very often a midwife will say, 'Doctor, why did you do that?' or 'I do not approve of this!' I think we need this. It is still fundamentally a question of character.[7]

It is also a question of title, since there is no generally accepted form of address for a midwife; one does not normally refer to 'Midwife Jones' the way one might refer to 'Nurse Jones'. Years ago midwives were given the honorary title of 'Mrs', i.e. 'Mrs Jones', but that has now lapsed in most areas. So midwives are called 'nurses', are administered by 'nursing officers' and are regarded by health authorities as part of the 'nursing staff'. None of this helps to maintain the image of midwifery as a separate profession.

The sort of character referred to by Professor Kloosterman is reflected also in the response of midwives to the erosion of their position and responsibilities. The bulk of the midwifery profession has been silent in the face of the rapid decline of home births, fragmentation of total care and reorganization of the Health Service administration, whereas in Denmark midwives struggling to retain their autonomy in childbirth decided in November 1973 to focus the nation's attention on their position by staging the first midwives' strike in the nation's history. They still attended births but they refused to fill out the lengthy forms on each birth required by the government.

In this country before 1948 midwives employed by the local authority booked their own patients and delivered them at home. Antenatal care was provided by the local authority clinic (doctor and midwife/ves) or in the patient's own home by her own midwife (GPs were involved only if the midwife needed help). If the GP was called to attend, then the midwife gave him a form from her triplicate form book which he then sent to the local authority who paid him for his services. The midwife kept a copy in her book, and her third copy was sent to the supervisor of midwives. Alternatively, the mother could be booked with her own GP or, if there were problems, booked for hospital.

In 1970 came the Peel report which recommended that 'facilities should be provided for 100 per cent hospital confinement'. The reason given for this recommendation was that hospitals were safer places for all women (there has been no evidence to support this claim, either at the time or since, and yet this assertion was put before the select committee[5] (para. 55) as the reason for pursuing the recommendations of the Peel report).

In 1974, the Health Service was reorganized and the newly formed Health Authorities took over the responsibilities of the local authorities. While GPs succeeded in retaining their position as independent practitioners, midwifery became an 'integrated' service, and the overall responsibility for the pregnant woman rested with 'the doctor' (either GP or hospital consultant) even if the midwives did most of the actual caring.

The effect of the implementation of the Peel report on the midwives in hospitals has been to increase dramatically their workload, which means effectively that they are seriously understaffed.[6] In 1979 a national survey was undertaken by the Nursing Education Research Unit, which involved, among other things, sending a questionnaire to all the midwives and obstetricians in sixty health districts and to a sample of general practitioners and health visitors. Most of the 2926 hospital midwives felt that there were falling and inadequate standards of patient care, both in general and in specific aspects of care, e.g. help with breast-feeding, and that there was inadequate cover on the wards particularly at night, both in terms of the actual numbers on duty and the availability of trained staff to take charge: there was often inadequate cover on the labour wards when they were busy; the midwives also complained of the effect that staff shortages had on the in-service training of pupil midwives (and student nurses) who were not properly instructed or supervised and were consequently lacking in confidence. They felt that there was an understandable reluctance on the part of newly qualified midwives to stay in the profession in view of the stresses which had to be endured. 'I can't begin to explain adequately: we frequently miss meal breaks because we are rushing from patient to patient in labour, trying to cope. . . .' Because of the pressure and nature of the work, there is no job satisfaction and most midwives feel exploited and overworked; consequently they leave to do other jobs, which exacerbates the situation. The midwives' workload was further increased as a result of the stepping up of obstetric technology, the so-called 'childbirth revolution' (*Sunday Times*, 13 October 1974). This automatically means more 'midwife hours' are needed: it has been shown that looking after mothers and babies following complicated births involves more work than looking after those with normal births; that episiotomies increase the workload, Caesarean sections double it, and nursing a baby in a special-care unit multiplies the workload by a factor of almost five.[8]

Much of what was inherent in midwifery practice (e.g. continuity of care), and particularly their independent practitioner status, has already been lost as far as the hospital midwife is concerned. The majority of doctors in a study carried out by Walker[9] thought they should 'take charge' if they arrived unexpectedly (i.e. had not been called in by the midwife) and the midwife was engaged in the process of a normal, uncomplicated delivery – traditionally her domain. Medicines and drugs given during a normal labour which *could* be prescribed by a midwife (on her own authority) are in many hospitals given only on medical prescription.

Community midwives also had their autonomy and authority further undermined by the Peel report. They lost 'their' mothers to the consultant obstetrician and their independence to the general practitioner. (This was and is still more than just encroachment on the management of normal labour, but extends to the antenatal care given to mothers.) A large proportion of midwives (90 per cent in hospital, 60 per cent in the community) who were consulted in the Chelsea survey[10] reported that abdominal examinations and examinations for oedema made by them were repeated by the doctor: this is a great waste of the midwife's time as well as of the doctor's, and calls into question the midwife's competence, undermining her responsibility and confidence as a practitioner, reducing her in some instances to 'little more than a chaperone for the medical staff'. The questionnaire tried to ascertain what proportion of midwives were ever given any responsibility for the total assessment and care of women at any antenatal visit. It was revealed that this was more likely to be the case if there was a midwives' clinic, which was held in the hospitals of twenty-two out of the sixty districts in the survey. Where these did exist, though, they were very small (6–12 patients) compared with 80–100 patients at the doctors' clinics, and it was likely that the doctors referred mothers to the midwives' clinic, rather than the other way round (as in Holland). Many of the hospital midwives in the survey specifically said that they would like to hold midwives' clinics and many of the heads of the midwifery service said that they would like to see the re-establishment of midwives' clinics. Over half the midwives in the survey said they would like to be able to take more responsibility and nearly half of those working in teaching hospitals felt that doctors were undertaking midwives' work.

Not surprisingly, community midwives too have begun to leave the profession: from 1974 (when the health services were reorganized) to 1978 the number of community midwives fell from 3625 to 2790, a drop of 23 per cent.[5] This erosion of status is now being reflected also in the recruitment of pupil midwives. The number of recruits has fallen progressively since the end of 1978.[11]

The Chelsea survey[6] found a shortfall of pupils ranging from 5.3 per cent to 25.5 per cent (a shortfall of midwives of between 7.5 per cent and 27 per cent), and the other main understaffed group – tutors – had a shortfall of 0 per cent to 23 per cent. The shortage of midwives will obviously have an effect on the quality of care which the service can provide. (In most of the regions to which the survey questionnaire was sent, it was the feeling of many of the community midwives that their standards of care were falling, that they did not have the time to attend antenatal clinics or private antenatal care in the home, and lacked time to spend with the mother and baby postnatally, particularly with regard to infant feeding. Many of them said that they had extra-heavy workloads to cover holidays, weekends and sickness, which entailed having to work overtime and do extra on-call duty, so reducing their job satisfaction as well as making them overtired and/or ill.)

The shortage of pupils will affect the service in years to come, and the shortage of tutors will affect the quality of education which pupils receive. The general shortage throughout the profession is likely to be made worse as the birthrate continues to rise, and simultaneously the midwife's working week is reduced from forty hours to thirty-seven and a half. The already understaffed hospital and community midwifery services will have a greater and greater workload and will be put under more and more pressure. This will surely become a vicious circle – as more midwives give up the struggle and leave the service, whilst others fail to join, the workload increases for those who remain and so on. . . . 'Midwifery used to be a vocation, a calling (we used to be on call twenty-four hours a day because we wanted to) now, sadly, it's a job.'[12]

This situation is not likely to improve until midwives are again allowed to do what they are trained to do, and can take up their role as independent practitioners and chief caretakers of the normal parturient woman. True caretaking, as far as the mother and midwife are concerned, means providing on-going antenatal and postnatal education and emotional support at all stages of the process (as well as the more obvious physical aspects of care) but this cannot be done unless it is possible to establish a relationship, which currently is only possible within the framework of community midwifery.

Hospital midwifery remains fragmented, the trend is to-wards specialization in one department – antenatal clinics, labour wards, postnatal wards and neonatal intensive-care units – an unnatural practice which is a source of considerable frustration to some midwives and more so to mothers who complain bitterly of long waits antenatally, seeing a different face at each visit, of lack of support in labour and conflicting advice postnatally. This fragmentation will not be improved by the introduction of 'specialist courses in labour ward prac-tice', as recommended in the Social Services Committee re-port.[5] Many midwives would in any case consider themselves by virtue of their midwifery training 'specialists' in labour ward practice[13] where birth is normal and their role is one of calm watchfulness, the minimum of interference and much emotional support. Where labour is not straightforward it is the province of the obstetrician. The majority of labours are normal and are not 'intensive-care situations', so that mid-wives should not be reduced to the 'specialization' of machine-minding!

It is surprising how many mothers, especially first-time mothers, are unaware of the fact that there is an alternative to hospital care. Some general practitioners – particularly if they are not on the obstetric list – automatically book their expectant patients for the hospital without explaining that there is another system of care available for those not considered to be at risk. Once the mother attends for her first (booking) visit in the hospital antenatal clinic, her case notes are filled in and she is assigned to one of the hospital consultants (who has been selected by her GP), it will be assumed that she is there from choice, and not that she is unaware that there *is* a choice.

In the majority of large maternity hospitals, the antenatal clinics are staffed by trained midwives who work only in the antenatal department, supervising the antenatal care, getting each woman ready to be seen by the doctor, and giving parentcraft or mothercraft classes. When the woman goes into labour, she is admitted to the labour ward and cared for by another, separate group of midwives who work only on the labour ward. Furthermore, if she is in labour in the middle of a duty 'shift', the midwife looking after her will change when the new shift comes on, so that the mother may have no continuity of care even in labour. When she has had her baby and is adjudged fit to leave, she goes to a postnatal ward where there is yet another contingent of midwives, nursery nurses and others, who work only with postnatal mothers and babies. When she leaves the hospital, she is visited at home until her baby is ten days old by a community midwife – yet another new face. The only 'through traffic' in all this is provided by the midwives in training, who are transferred from department to department within the hospital as their training progresses – but the chances of their following a mother through each 'fragment' of her total care are very remote.

In complete contrast, the woman who has no need of the specialist care which the consultant unit provides can be cared for by a general practitioner and a midwife, and delivered either at home or in a general practitioner unit, either inside or outside a consultant unit (i.e. a maternity home/outlying GP unit, or a GP unit within the larger maternity hospital). If the woman's own GP does not provide obstetric care, or will not take on 'first-time' mothers, the woman is perfectly entitled to register with any other GP of her choice who will agree to take her for the duration of her pregnancy, labour and puerperium – six weeks after delivery. This does not mean that she leaves her own family GP's list, but merely that she goes elsewhere for her maternity care. The majority of community midwives are now group-attached rather than geographically based, that is, they care for all pregnant patients of a particular GP regardless of where the patients live.

When a mother finds, or is already registered, with a GP who will care for her during pregnancy, the midwife will receive an official request from the GP to see the mother. This first booking visit, which takes place in the mother's home, can and should take at least one and a half hours during which time the woman's history is taken, the case notes are filled in and the foundations of the mother–midwife relationship are laid. The midwife continues to see the mother at the same regular intervals as the GP, sometimes with him and sometimes in the mother's home. Apart from any more structured antenatal classes the mother may obtain at health centre clinics or from National Childbirth Trust teachers, the midwife provides informal antenatal education where appropriate through her visits during the pregnancy. When the mother goes into labour, she rings the midwife's coordinating office (or, if she has been told to do so, the midwife's home): either her own midwife or her midwife's partner, should the first be off duty, will talk to her and either go to see her at home or if more appropriate arrange to meet her at the clinic or hospital.

The same applies if the mother goes into labour at 'night' (6 p.m.–8.30 a.m.), except that the number of possible alternatives to the mother's own midwife is slightly increased since the 'on-call' duty is usually shared on a rota system by an average of four midwives, one of whom will cover at night for all the practices to which she and the other midwives are attached: even so, it is likely that the mother will have met all of the very small number of midwives who might attend her labour. If it is her own midwife who is called to her in labour, she will remain with the mother right through the labour regardless of how long it is, so that she has continuous support throughout. The GP is informed that this patient is in labour, and informed again when she is in the second stage; but he does not usually attend unless the midwife specifically requests his presence because there are problems. It is the midwife who delivers the mother (unless there *are* problems) whether or not the doctor is present.

(It is of interest to note that in countries where the labour and delivery are in the hands of skilled midwives, whether at home or in hospital, the perinatal mortality rate is very low, e.g. Sweden and Finland, who have 100 per cent hospital confinement, and Holland, which has 50 per cent hospital confinement. In those countries where obstetricians have taken over normal labours and deliveries and the midwife has either ceased to exist or has been relegated to the status of obstetric nurse (as in the USA), perinatal mortality has been much slower to fall.)

Both during and after the birth the parents' wishes can be respected, and the baby can stay with the mother and feed when it is ready. The midwife is not constrained to follow unthinking rules and regulations as her hospital counterpart may be. She will not leave the new family until she is satisfied that all is well, and she will return a few hours later to check again and to answer any questions. During the whole postnatal period, which can if necessary be anything up to twenty-eight days, the same midwife will call (apart from off-duty days) so that the mother has her help and guidance at a period when she is emotionally very vulnerable, and has this from someone she already knows and trusts.

This is particularly important if the mother is breast-feeding: it takes time, patience and continual encouragement to help a first-time mother or a mother breast-feeding for the first time to succeed. More mothers give up as a result of destroyed confidence (through conflicting or misleading information) and sore nipples (due to incorrect positioning of the baby on the breast) than ever give up due to 'insufficient milk' – a reason which is often given. . . . In Third World countries, where there is no safe alternative to breast-feeding, but where one might have expected more mothers to have insufficient milk through their own malnourished state, the number of those mothers with lactation failure is surprisingly low. A survey conducted by Dr David Morley in a rural Nigerian village found less than 1 per cent of mothers with serious problems. Between 2 per cent and 3 per cent had temporary trouble due to illness, but still managed to breast-feed their babies for six months. 'In urban areas of the Third World, figures are hard to come by: Nestlé estimate that perhaps 5 per cent of mothers would have difficulty. Doctors confirm this as the likely maximum figure.'[14]

The personal and continuous care which a community mid-wifery service can provide seems not only to produce better results in terms of outcome, particularly for babies when low-risk groups are compared (Goodlin,[15] Taylor et al.,[16] Mehl et al.[17]), but also provide greater psychological and emotional satisfaction for mothers (Kitzinger,[18] Goldthorpe and Richman,[19] AIMS[20]).

The 'recommendations' made by the Social Services Committee on the subject of midwives and their training (pp. 71–9) make it clear that the committee is aware the country is very short of midwives and that the situation is likely to get worse unless changes are made. It also seems to recognize that this state of affairs is largely due to the fact that the midwife has 'less opportunity to practice the job she expects and has been trained to do' and has suffered a 'loss of personal status'. It therefore recommends that midwives should be helped to regain their former status (para. 249) and that 'every effort is made to re-establish midwifery as a profession that offers attractive prospects to young women'. These statements are seemingly incompatible with many of the other recommendations made, in particular (para. 523–10) that 'an increased number of mothers should he delivered in large units'. This recommendation has its origins in the Peel report which, the committee was informed by the DHSS, provided the basis of present policy. As Marjorie Tew points out, 'They were not apparently told that it is now generally acknowledged that the Peel Committee had no evidence whatsoever to justify its claim [that hospitals were safer], nor has any been found since.'[21]

The Social Services Committee is still hoping to keep the maternity service on course for 100 per cent hospital confinements, under the increasing control of hospital consultants who are used to having the service revolve around them rather than the patients.[22] 'The delivery should be exactly as the *woman* desires – but we all know this is impossible in a hospital. Hospitals are self-serving' (Michael Whitt, MD).[23] If this recommendation is implemented, it will mean that the service continues to be centred on the 10 per cent of abnormal births without regard for the implications of hospital confinement on those who neither need nor want it. Chalmers, Oakley and MacFarlane have recently urged 'that the very normality of most childbearing women means that they should be protected from the adverse effects of policies formulated through concern for the minority'.[24]

The committee's proposals concerning the place of birth imply a continued fragmentation of care for mothers and a continued reduction in the number of community midwives. They will do nothing to improve the image of the midwifery profession (whose members are to be discouraged from pursuing independent practitioner status, para. 225), or to alleviate the staffing shortages.

The committee proposed to make good the midwifery staffing deficiencies by the employment of nonqualified staff and also by mounting a national campaign to recruit newly qualified nurses into midwifery. Nonqualified staff will be able to relieve the pressure only where it is caused by midwives having to undertake nonmidwifery duties – e.g. emptying bins, giving out meals, etc. They will make no impression where the problem is actual shortage of trained midwives to care for the mothers directly. Recruiting newly qualified nurses at a time when there is a reduced number qualifying (because of the drop in recruits into nursing in 1977) is irresponsible, as general hospitals will then lose out: it is a waste of three years' expensive nursing training and will simply perpetuate the problem of the 'nursing approach' to midwifery discussed earlier.

The committee does, however, mention in passing increasing 'direct entry' into midwifery (para. 238). This, combined with a lengthened and redesigned training course (para. 243 and 244) may be the salvation of the midwifery profession. If the present two-year training course were extended to three years and modelled on Denmark's training scheme where the entire first year is spent becoming conversant with normal births, the end result might be more qualified midwives in possession of not only a certificate but also an 'intuitive confidence in the process of childbearing, as opposed to a pathological perception'.[25] Such midwives would be more likely to demand the freedom to practise independently as the Midwives Act (1951) entitles them to do, and would want to assume their traditional role as caretakers of normal parturient women. This would be most easily achieved by 'allowing' more births to take place outside hospitals (homes, GP units) managed by midwives and not obstetricians.

Facilities for normal family birth (not necessarily at home), into which full intensive care can be injected at a moment's notice, are what parents, midwives and child psychiatrists want. There are vocal and determined parents voicing their criticisms [of the present system]. Already a few have turned their backs on the service and to continue to ignore this is to court disaster.[22]

For those women who need the facilities which obstetricians can offer, much could still be done to improve the quality and continuity of their care. Caroline Flint has described a scheme whereby continuity of care could be achieved within a hospital setting.[26] Its limitations include the fact that it would not be appropriate to all women (even within the hospital) and that it does not extend the continuity into the postnatal period, but it is a vast improvement on what is currently offered in the majority of hospitals.

As Pamela Slack has pointed out,[22] there is a fundamental organizational problem which must be faced if mothers are to receive the service they want and midwives are to provide the service they are trained to provide; it may be that, as central government continues to act as if unaware of the implications of the current situation, the future of midwifery may depend not only on how effectively the midwife stands her ground, but ultimately upon the determination of mothers themselves in exercising their right to give birth where and how they wish.

Appendix 1

An outline of the process of labour

Countdown to labour

Low backache, general feelings of heaviness in vagina and pelvic floor, menstrual-like discomfort with strong pregnancy (Braxton Hicks) contractions. A burst of 'nesting' activity – washing floors, clearing out cupboards, etc. Very often the lower bowel is completely emptied, due to either loose or small, frequent bowel motions.

The beginnings of labour

1. A 'show' – thick, jelly-like mucus, which may be light-brownish, purply-red or streaked with bright red. It is usually an indication that the cervix has started to dilate and detach itself partly from the membranes. It may precede the onset of the labour by a few days or a few hours, and sometimes it is passed after regular contractions have started. Occasionally it may be dislodged by a vigorous vaginal examination, and in this situation the fresh blood streaking may be slightly heavier; there should, however, be no real bleeding – if there is seek medical attention immediately.

A show is not always reliable as an indication that labour is about to start, and unless the mother is worried about its colour, it is not an event that needs to be reported to the midwife/doctor/hospital.

2. Prior to the onset of labour the baby's chin is in most cases tucked into his/her chest, so that the top/back of the head fits snugly into the cervix. When this happens, the fluid in front of the head is cut off from the remainder of the amniotic fluid and becomes known as the forewaters, the remainder being known as the hindwaters. This system reduces the pressure which is applied to the forewaters by the contracting uterus, and helps to keep them intact despite strong contractions. Thus, the closed system of amniotic fluid can continue to perform its physiological function in labour – that of equalizing the pressure applied to all parts of the baby, its cord and placenta – in most cases throughout the greater part of the first stage.

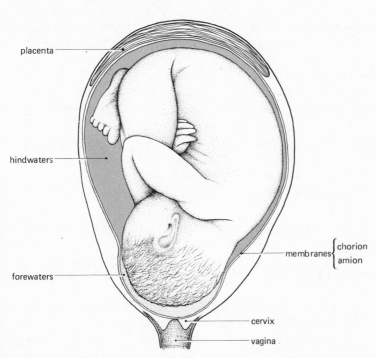

However, the membranes may rupture before the contractions start. This is more common when the baby is lying in a posterior position. The 'break' in the bag of waters may be behind the baby's head and therefore it trickles out slowly – a 'hindwater leak'. The easiest way for the mother to decide whether she is leaking urine or liquor (amniotic fluid) is to empty her bladder deliberately, put on a sanitary towel and see whether or not she continues to get wet. If in doubt, she should ring the hospital/midwife. The midwife may test the fluid with litmus paper (liquor is alkaline and will turn red litmus paper blue, whilst urine is commonly acid, and will turn blue litmus paper red). The newer alternative is nitrazene sticks which turn from yellow to black in the presence of amniotic fluid. Sometimes the membranes in front of the baby's head rupture. In this case, the liquor will gush out more obviously (anything from half to one and a half cupfuls – just that which is 'trapped' in front of the baby's head). This is more likely to occur after the contractions have started, but may be early on in the labour. If it happens as the first event, contractions usually start fairly quickly afterwards, unlike those in the case of the hindwater leak.

In both instances, the midwife/hospital should be informed. The main reason for this is that the longer the interval between membrane rupture and delivery, the greater the risk of infection of the amniotic fluid. Doctors vary in their view as to how long it is safe to wait for contractions to start after the membranes rupture before they give intravenous oxytocin in a drip, but most will give prophylactic antibiotics after 12–24 hours.

The other reason for reporting a rupture of the membranes is so that a vaginal examination can be carried out to exclude cord prolapse if an abdominal examination shows that the baby's head is not engaged.

3.   Contractions rarely start 'out of the blue' – there is usually some warning that things are about to happen. Much more commonly the woman may 'miss' the very beginning of labour in the sense of knowing the precise time that contractions

begin. The unseen physiological preparation for labour which takes place in the woman's body is a gradual process. Over the weeks and months, the Braxton Hicks contractions slowly become more noticeable and stronger, and may begin the process of thinning out and shortening the cervix before labour starts in earnest. Quite often this beginning of labour is discounted as just another bout of Braxton Hicks contractions, until the realization that these are occurring at regular intervals. It is, however, not uncommon for a woman to have one or more episodes of regular contractions towards the end of pregnancy which are fairly weak and do not become progressively longer and stronger, and then cease altogether, after having lasted as long as four hours.

'True' labour contractions therefore may be recognized by the fact that not only do they occur at regular intervals, but as time goes by the intervals reduce and the contractions feel stronger (and are in fact dilating the cervix). They may begin at intervals of 20–30 minutes and last 30 seconds or so, but gradually increase to 5–10 minutes with about 45–50-second duration, and towards the end of the first stage they may be between 2–4 minutes apart, lasting 50–60 seconds. As the second stage approaches, the contractions may in some cases occur every $1\frac{1}{2}$–2 minutes, and last 60–90 seconds so that the woman may feel that they are continuous.

Sometimes the contractions may die down for a short period before the second stage starts, and when they resume, they are different in quality as the expulsive urge builds up. Sometimes, the first and second stages seem to overlap, and the urge to push may begin before the cervix is fully dilated. This transitional phase of labour may be characterized by irritability, disorientation, nausea, vomiting, backache, a trancelike state in which the woman feels rooted to the spot and any movement requires enormous effort (onlookers may think she is asleep), shaking of legs and/or whole body, cold feet, and a gradual building up of rectal pressure as the baby's head follows the sacral curve down, round and forwards. She may also find she is 'catching' her breath or grunting with contractions.

In most cases, second-stage contractions build up gradually both in quality and efficiency: the expulsive urge usually comes at the height of the contraction, not at the beginning (it may recur in a wavelike fashion within one contraction). In some women the expulsive sensation is mild or absent, in some totally overwhelming, and in the majority it is experienced as a powerful surge of energy. As the baby's head starts to stretch the vagina and perineum, the mother may experience a hot, stretching, burning sensation round the entrance to the vagina, which reaches its peak as the widest part of the baby's head is born (crowning).

Often there is a pause (1–2 minutes) after the head is born while the final contraction is awaited – the contraction which will deliver the baby's body. As the baby emerges, it will follow the continuation of the pelvic curve onto the mother's abdomen with her help, or the help of the birth attendant.

For a further description of labour, see S. Kitzinger, *The Experience of Childbirth*, Penguin, 3rd edn, 1972; and S. Kitzinger, *Birth at Home*, Oxford University Press, 1979.

Appendix 2

Arranging a home birth

The Midwives Act of 1936, which later became consolidated into the Midwives Act of 1951, made it compulsory for local authorities to provide sufficient midwives to attend women confined at home in their area. This act has not been repealed, and the obligation was passed to the Area Health Authorities when in 1974 they took over from the local authorities. Furthermore, the Central Midwives Board dictates that a midwife called to a woman in labour *must* attend. Social services departments are similarly obliged to provide home helps for a two-week period following a home delivery and longer if the GP considers it necessary. In 1978, Dr David Ennals, then the Minister of Health and Social Security, was quoted in *The Times* as saying,

It would be wrong for the Government to insist that mothers who want to have their babies at home should have them in hospital. I have to make it quite clear that if a woman chooses to have her delivery at home, despite arguments against it, the Area Health Authorities should ensure that the services necessary to make home delivery as safe as possible are provided.[1]

More recently Patrick Jenkin (currently Secretary of State for Social Services) is on record as saying, 'we would not necessarily agree [with the Short report] that births at home should be phased out further. . . . My view, quite clearly, is that where a mother reasonably insists on having her baby at home, I expect health authorities to provide a domiciliary service that is as safe as circumstances permit.'[2]

Mothers therefore do still have the right to choose to have their babies at home and the right to expect that there will be sufficient midwives, doctors and emergency services (flying squads) to ensure their safety as far as possible. No mother can be given a guarantee of safety for herself or her baby, irrespective of where she delivers: women with identifiable risk factors (see pages 28–31) are statistically more likely to run into difficulties at home, but that does not mean that this is inevitable. (It does depend, of course, on what the risk factor is.) In the absence of definite contraindications in the present pregnancy or previous labour, a woman who wants to deliver at home can aim to do so, bearing in mind that she can be transferred to hospital if the need arises. It would be unwise for a woman to decide that she will have her baby at home *whatever* happens, since it is impossible to know for sure in advance what will happen in the course of the labour: this however is an argument for flexibility in attitude, not an argument for 100 per cent hospital confinement. In England and Wales in 1970, there were only four infant deaths per thousand at home, compared with a figure of seventeen per thousand overall, and it is probable that those deaths which occurred at home would have occurred irrespective of where the baby was born. What is more, the figures for perinatal deaths at home include all deaths of babies born outside hospital: into this category come all concealed pregnancies, premature and precipitate deliveries, etc., which were in fact booked for hospital delivery – or not booked at all. As the number of *planned* home deliveries with low perinatal mortality rate falls, the high perinatal mortality rate of the unplanned group will progressively distort the composite figure, and make it appear that these deaths at home are much more common than they really are. This point was aptly made by Dr Bull in the *Observer* (29 June 1980), criticizing the article in the same paper on 15 June 1980, entitled 'Danger at home for new babies'. Mothers may simply be told that deaths at home are 'on the increase', or that 'it is becoming more dangerous to have a baby at home', without any further explanation. It has even been suggested that 'home delivery is the earliest form of child abuse',[3] or that legislation should be introduced to prevent women from taking action which could damage their babies.[4] Such suggestions beg the question of legislation to prevent cigarette smoking, or crossing the road away from a crossing – activities both potentially much more dangerous, but where the right to choose and the right to take calculated risks go unquestioned. . . . Of much more relevance is the sad fact that although there may be no reason why a mother should not give birth at home, there is an increasing shortage of midwives and doctors who are sufficiently competent and confident to attend her in such cases, with the result that some areas do not 'offer' home birth facilities and women have to struggle to get what they want.

The commonest way to obtain professional attendance at a home birth is to seek the services of an NHS general practitioner and midwife team. This usually means that the mother visits the GP with whom she is registered and discusses the matter with him: if he agrees, all is well. If he is unwilling or unable to help, then the mother has the right to transfer to another doctor for the period of the pregnancy, birth and puerperium (six weeks following the birth). Her own GP may suggest a colleague, otherwise she may learn from friends, organizations and support groups such as the Society for the Support of Home Confinements, from the local community midwife supervisor or the Family Practitioner Committee (see the telephone directory for addresses), the name of a GP who is likely to be amenable.

A GP who is willing to accept the mother for a home birth will have one or more midwives attached to his practice and one of them will be assigned to the mother for the duration of her pregnancy and labour and for up to one month afterwards if necessary. Although the midwife may carry out most of the work, it will be the GP in this case who has overall responsibility. The mother is under no legal obligation to have the services of a doctor, and if she cannot find one willing to accept her for a home delivery, she can obtain the services of a midwife on her own, either a private midwife or an NHS community midwife. The services of the NHS midwife are obtained by contacting the District Nursing Officer, or, if there is one, the Nursing Officer for Community Midwifery. The midwife provided (and the DHA have a duty to provide one) will be acting as a practitioner in her own right, and will be responsible for the mother's antenatal care, delivery and care after the birth. If the midwife feels that it is inadvisable for the mother to be delivered at home, she may say so in writing to her superiors, but she still has a duty to continue her attendance on the mother. Junor and Monaco[5] comment that the Society for the Support of Home Confinements know of no instance where the procedure of requesting a midwife from the AHA has failed to produce satisfactory results. They add, 'Remember that it is possible to get a home birth anywhere, despite initial, sometimes adamant denials to the contrary by some AHAs.'

The services of a private midwife can be obtained by applying to a private nursing agency, the Royal College of Midwives or possibly the Association of Radical Midwives. The midwife is again acting as a practitioner in her own right and has overall responsibility for the mother's care. She will probably make her own arrangements with a doctor, on whom she can call in an emergency.

Useful publications

Marianne Monaco and Vicky Junor, *Home Birth Handbook*. BIJA Press, 1980. Obtainable from 47 Valence Road, Lewes, Sussex, or Manor House, Thelnetham, Nr Diss, Norfolk IP22 1JZ

Sheila Kitzinger, *Birth at Home*, Oxford University Press, 1979

Useful addresses

Society for the Support of Home Confinements, c/o Margaret Whyte, 17 Laburnum Ave, Durham

Association of Radical Midwives, Lakefield, 8A The Drive, Wimbledon, London SW19

Association for the Improvement of the Maternity Services, 19 Allerton Grange Crescent, Chapel Allerton, Leeds LS17 5LN

Home birth

A true comparison between home and institutional delivery will never be achieved until it is possible to study outcomes such as the long-term quality of births in terms of physical, psychological and mental health, the benefits to the mother of relief of pain or anxiety, the long-term benefits in terms of incidence of complications such as prolapse, urinary incontinence and other similar measures.[6]

In the meantime the arguments surrounding home births centre on safety and emotional wellbeing, sometimes as if these two factors were mutually exclusive. Most of the points raised in this section have already been discussed in detail earlier in the book and what follows is a summary of the advantages and disadvantages of both hospital and home deliveries.

Hospital delivery: the advantages

1.   The most obvious and undisputed advantage is the immediate availability, in a good hospital, of the necessary equipment and expertise to cope with difficulties and emergencies which may arise in labour. Any woman who has good reason to anticipate problems in her labour or with her newborn baby would be wise to elect to give birth in a suitably equipped and staffed hospital.

2.   There may be *social advantages* where a mother's domestic situation or home surroundings are not suitable. The most important social factor at home is that the mother has suf-

ficient help after the baby is born. The fact that the hous
has only cold water on tap or that the toilet is at the bottom
of the garden are not necessarily reasons for advising against
home confinement, provided there is sufficient *willing* help
but it may be that the mother feels that she would be better
off using the facilities provided in hospital.

3.   *Psychological advantages* Women have been told repeat
edly that birth in hospital is safer for them all. The fact that
this statement is not supported by any evidence (see page 26
will not stop a substantial number of women from believing
it, and it would be just as bad to oblige a woman who had no
anticipated medical need of hospital facilities to give birth a
home as it would be to insist that she went into hospital. In
all labour, peace of mind is an important factor (see page 38
and a woman should be able to give birth in the place in
which she feels safe and secure – which for a proportion of
women will mean in a hospital.

There may also be some advantage to be gained from the
contacts made by the newly delivered mother with others in
the same position. Friendships made in this situation may be
valuable and supportive both in hospital and when the moth
ers go home.

Hospital delivery: the disadvantages

1.   The mother is usually subjected to all the procedures
which are routine in a hospital, regardless of her individual
needs.

2.   Friends and relations are greatly restricted in the support
they can give the mother, both during the labour and once
the baby is born.

3.   She is more likely to be subjected to the whims of indi
vidual members of staff who have a 'territorial advantage'.

4.   She is more likely to be subjected to unnecessary inter
ference simply because the facilities are there (see page 33).

5.   She is more likely to be given drugs as a 'first resort'
rather than as a 'last resort' (see page 98).

.   She is much less free to respond to her own feelings about what is right for her, what she wears, eats, drinks, the position he adopts during the first and second stages, where and how he actually gives birth, what happens to the baby and cord fter birth, when she feeds the baby, etc. (all these aspects re covered in the main part of the book).

Home delivery: the disadvantages

The reason most often given by professionals for opposing ome birth is that it is 'not safe' or 'not as safe as hospital'. They do not mean that more babies (or mothers) die at home, ince the figures for perinatal mortality for babies born at ome are very much lower than for those born in hospital,[7] particularly when one considers those babies whose mothers were actually selected for a home confinement. They mean hat if things should go wrong, the facilities are not available t home to put them right. Firstly, this assumes that if things o wrong in hospital it is always possible to put them right. Unfortunately, there are certain unpredictable disasters which befall mothers and babies, which simply cannot be put right, o matter where they take place (e.g. amniotic fluid embolism n the mother, or congenital malformations in the baby which re incompatible with life, such as anencephaly), and no nother can be given an assurance of absolute safety simply because she is confined in hospital. The concept of 'absolute afety' in childbirth is illusory and should be accepted as such by mothers and professionals alike, yet this was a phrase actually used by the Short Committee in their published report on 'Perinatal and Neonatal Mortality'.

It also assumes that midwives are ill-equipped to deal with any unpredictable emergencies arising at home. In fact, community midwives attending home deliveries are not only rained, as are all midwives, in the management for example of a heavy post-delivery bleed (postpartum haemorrhage), or a baby who does not breathe immediately, but have at their disposal the same drugs and equipment as their hospital counterparts, e.g. ergometrine and syntometrine (which stimulate he uterus to contract), portable oxygen, face mask, mucus

extraction catheter, cardiac and respiratory stimulants and th
necessary needles and syringes. A complete list of equipmen
is given later in this section, page 231. The midwife at home
also has – or should have – the facility to call on a mobil
obstetric emergency service, previously known as the 'flying
squad', should the need arise, or to arrange to transport th
mother to hospital by car or ambulance if she feels the mothe
may need the help of an obstetrician or her baby the help o
a paediatrician.

With proper selection (see pages 28–31) at the beginning o
the pregnancy, revised if necessary during the pregnancy a
a result of the good antenatal care the mother should hav
received, the incidence of avoidable mishaps at home birth
is very low. (A study of 5000 home births in Holland showed
that of the few deaths which occurred in the group, non
could have been prevented had the birth taken place in hos
pital[8] and the British Birth Survey (1970)[7] has shown tha
babies born in hospital are five times more likely to hav
breathing difficulties than those born at home.)

Finally, there is the question of the degree of risk. Man
aspects of our lives involve the taking of calculated risks
Every time we cross a road or drive a car, or take a seat in
plane, we are taking a calculated risk. If there were not oc
casions on which we were able to put our trust in ourselve
or in someone else, life would come to a standstill. Deciding
to embark on a pregnancy involves the taking of a calculated
risk; so too does deciding where and how to give birth. Every
mother, consciously or unconsciously, makes a decision which
involves the taking of risks. If she allows herself to be confined
in hospital, without discussing the reasons for it, she is taking
the risk that her advisers may not be considering her individ
ual needs but merely following policy, and, once in hospital
that the risk of unnecessary interference is greater than the
potential benefits conferred on her by actually being there. I
she consciously makes a choice, then she must have con
sidered the advantages and disadvantages of her choice. If she
decides that she wants her baby born at home, then, as with
hospital, she has adjudged that in her circumstances the ben

fits for her of her chosen place of confinement outweigh the hazards. All that professionals and others can do is to make sure that the mother has as much accurate information at her disposal as possible so that she makes an informed choice, since it is she who bears the child and copes in the long term with the consequences of the decisions taken around the time of birth.

Home delivery: the advantages

1.   Antenatally, the mother is likely to have been cared for by one GP and midwife, and to have met the other midwives in the group, so that she has had continuity of care and a chance to talk to and develop a trusting relationship with the people who will help her during labour.

2.   When antenatal visits take place at home, the mother is relaxed and other children in the family have a chance to get to know the midwife and become involved in the preparations for their new sister or brother.

3.   There is much less disturbance in the lives of the mother's other children if the birth of the new baby does not coincide with the disappearance of the mother. Jealousy is more likely to be avoided if the only problem the other child or children have to cope with is the arrival of the baby.

4.   The expectant parents are not faced with the need to 'decide' when labour has really started and when to go into hospital; the midwife can be contacted by telephone and she will visit the mother at home.

5.   If labour starts slowly, the midwife may leave the couple or family for a period, returning when either she or the mother feels her presence is necessary.

6.   Once labour is established, the midwife stays with the mother until the baby is delivered, thus providing continuous emotional and practical support.

7.   There are no admission procedures and no forms for the mother to complete. Perineal shaving is rarely performed at

home and enemas or suppositories are given only if the need is indicated.

8.　The mother can choose what she wears for labour.

9.　The mother can move around during her labour, experimenting with different positions to increase her comfort.

10.　She may eat or drink, as she feels inclined.

11.　There is no audience at her birth, except of her own choosing, and her other children may be present if she desires.

12.　She is able to use the breathing and relaxation technique she has learnt with the understanding and support of the midwife, who is much more likely to be familiar with the sort of antenatal instruction the mother has received.

13.　Drugs are likely to be administered only at the request of the mother, or if the midwife feels them to be essential.

14.　The mother is much less likely to have her labour interfered with or actively 'managed'.

15.　Familiar surroundings and an atmosphere of calm are likely to assist the mother in relaxing and tuning in to her labour so that she can follow her own body rhythms.

16.　The midwife and doctor are guests in the mother's home, and throughout labour attention is focused upon her and her individual wishes are respected.

17.　The mother can decide the place and position for the second stage: there is no necessity for her to give birth in or on a bed if she would rather be on the floor, or to give birth sitting or lying if she would rather be squatting, standing or on all fours.

18.　Episiotomy (a subject that the mother can discuss with the midwife beforehand) is much less likely to be performed at a home birth. There is usually no arbitrary time limit imposed on labours at home, and the second stage can be allowed to progress at its own pace, provided mother and baby show no signs of distress.

19. The way in which the baby is treated once it is born is again up to the mother, and she can hold it and feed it when she feels she wants to, without asking permission.

20. The baby's father is able to play a more positive role and will be more confident in his attitude towards his wife at home. He can wear his own clothes and sit beside or behind his wife, holding her in his arms if that seems appropriate. He may even help deliver the baby if he wants to and if the mother and midwife have no objection.

21. The mother at no point surrenders her responsibility for herself, her labour, her family or her newborn baby. Feeling close to and learning about caring for a new baby is easier when the mother can play it by ear rather than by prescribed routines.

22. Breast-feeding is easier to establish at home. Nonlimited sucking time and intervals help to minimize engorgement and promote a good milk supply. Night feeding is much less tiring if the mother can simply take the baby into bed with her and lie down to feed it when it cries, thus avoiding the necessity of being fully awakened several times a night, and there is no one to put a spanner in the works by giving the baby a bottle feed without the mother's permission. Thirty per cent of babies are still being bottle fed by hospital staff without their mother's consent, according to a survey published in the April 1981 issue of *Parents Magazine*.

The advice given to the mother on all aspects of the post-natal period, but in particular on breast-feeding, is likely to be consistent: she will not be bombarded with conflicting information by whichever nurses or midwives happen to be on duty.

23. The baby is much less likely to acquire an infection at home. The baby's skin is rapidly colonized by the harmless germs which share the home with his/her parents and brothers

and sisters. Hospital staff, on the other hand, have to be constantly aware of the dangers of crossinfection. The greatest problem of crossinfection in maternity units is presented by harmful strains of a bacteria which is known as staphylococcus aureous (yellow, pus-forming bacteria). Usually, such bacteria are relatively harmless, but penicillin-resistant strains have developed in hospital due to their continual exposure to antibiotics in powders and sprays, and these penicillin-resistant strains are usually the organisms responsible for epidemics in nurseries and maternity units.

24.   Postnatal blues (*not* postnatal depression) are much less likely following a home birth, as the mother does not have to cope with a sharp change in her environment (going home from hospital), or suddenly take over the total responsibility for her baby from others. Neither does she have to share the early days with strange women and their babies.

It can be seen from this list that for an expectant mother who is not in a category of increased risk, who is within reach of emergency facilities, and who is in the care of a skilled and confident midwife, that there are considerable advantages in staying at home for the birth of her baby if that is what she wants to do. There is more to childbirth than simply the production of a live baby and live mother. For many women, how the baby is born is equally important. Giving birth is now an event which for most women will occur only once or twice in a lifetime, and it is a very significant experience which cannot be shrugged off with 'better luck next time' if it is not the clichéd happy event. The mother's perception of herself and her child may be greatly affected by the circumstances and atmosphere surrounding the birth, and by the care, consideration and respect she received from her attendants.

The actual obstetric details may be less important than the way the mother *feels* about the birth. A mother who has had a perfectly straightforward labour and delivery but who was frightened, neglected, spoken to unkindly, or given drugs against her wishes, may remember the experience as a nightmare, whereas a mother who has had a benignly abnormal, possibly long and tedious labour, but who was supported and encouraged, given explanations and not left alone, may remember it as 'all right'. The experience of childbirth, whether good or bad, is not forgotten, although it may be buried, and may colour the mother's thinking and relationship with her child and the rest of her family for many years.

Planning a home birth

At some point during the latter part of the pregnancy, the midwife who has been caring for the mother antenatally will visit her at home to discuss the necessary arrangements for the birth. The most important thing the midwife will want to know is that the mother has sufficient help and support in the house for at least two weeks after the birth – either the father, another relative or friend(s). It is also important to ensure that the mother has the means to heat the room in which the baby will be born, and the room(s) in which it will be after the birth. There is no need for the room to be heated during labour, until the delivery is imminent, but thereafter it should be possible to maintain a temperature of 70–75 degrees Fahrenheit. A room thermometer, bought or borrowed, is thus a necessary piece of equipment. The room in which the delivery is planned should be reasonably clean and the midwife will need some cleaned surface – table, chest of drawers, dressing table or floor – on which to place her equipment. She will also need a good light in order to see what she is doing: this means either a strong overhead light (100-watt bulb) or, if the mother requests dim lighting, an alternative light source such as an anglepoise or adjustable table lamp. Although it is not necessary for the mother to deliver in a bed (a firm sofa, chaise longue, or the floor will do), the majority of women do get onto the bed for the actual birth, in which case the mattress needs to be fairly firm, or made firm by placing a board underneath it. It is very difficult for the midwife to attend to the baby's head and face when it is born, check for a cord round the neck or guide the shoulders safely over the perineum without causing tears if the mother's lower half is submerged in a feather mattress. (In these circumstances a left lateral position might be preferable.)

A mattress will require some means of protection, particularly once the waters break, and it is advisable to place layers of newspaper and/or a plastic or rubber sheet over the mattress and under the bottom sheet from about 36–7 weeks of the pregnancy – this advice could be given to all pregnant women, as the waters commonly break during a time when the mother is in bed – particularly if this is the first indication that labour has started or is about to start. Old linen which can be used for drawsheets, and if necessary thrown away afterwards, also helps to protect the bed and bedsheets both during and after labour.

The midwife must have easy access to a telephone either in the house or in a neighbour's, to enable her to keep in touch with the mother during early labour, to inform the GP of progress, or to summon help in an emergency.

The midwife will give the mother a list of additional articles which need to be available, and these will vary according to what the midwife's own delivery bag contains in any given region. The list will include:

1. A large cardboard box for all the rubbish, wrapped in newspaper, including the placenta which the midwife takes away with her.

2. Plenty of newspaper for protecting carpet and working surfaces, and for wrapping rubbish.

3. Water. The midwife will need to wash her hands, scrub her nails and dilute her lotions, as well as swabbing the mother's perineum prior to and after the delivery. If there is hot and cold running water in the bathroom on the same floor as the delivery room, the midwife can wash her hands there. Otherwise she will need a large bowl in the room, together with soap, nailbrush and towel (if she does not provide these herself). She will need cooled boiled water to dilute lotions and to swab the baby's eyes if necessary. Hot water will also be needed to fill hot water bottles, one of which will go into

the baby's sleeping container (crib, Moses basket, carrycot, drawer, etc.), to warm the receiving blanket, clothes and the mattress. Other than this, boiling water is required only for making tea or other hot drinks. Vast quantities of boiled water, beloved of television dramas, are required only if there is no hot running water in the house or the midwife has to sterilize instruments – very unlikely in areas with a central sterile supply department.

4.   A measuring jug for measuring blood loss after delivery, unless one is contained in the delivery pack.

5.   A bottle of antiseptic, if the midwife does not provide one.

6.   A couple of bowls for lotions – again, if not provided by the midwife.

7.   A thermometer and a small jar in which to keep it, unless the midwife has her own.

8.   A bedpan or a chamber pot or a toilet on the same floor as the delivery room. A child's potty will do, or a bedpan may be borrowed from the Red Cross if the midwife does not plan to bring one with her.

9.   Disposable enemas. These are either provided by the midwife should the need arise, or obtained on prescription from a chemist.

10.   Woolly socks and a cardigan, for warmth in labour if necessary.

After the delivery

The mother will need soap, flannel, towel, toothbrush and hair brush, either for a bed bath or to use in the bathroom.

She will need a clean nightdress and clean bed linen, including a clean drawsheet, several dozen sanitary pads, and the means for keeping them in place.

The baby will need

1.   A receiving blanket (any piece of clean old towel big enough to wrap the baby in straight after delivery).

2.   Two full-size hot water bottles for warming the receiving blanket, the cot and clothes. These are removed before the baby is put in the cot, so they do not need to have covers. (If bottles are placed in the cot with the baby at any point they will of course need to have covers.)

3.   Baby bath or washing-up bowl. This is optional: babies do not actually need baths to keep them clean. There are alternatives.

4.   Soap or other proprietary cleaner, cotton wool ($1/2$ lb) for the cleaning, and a towel for the baby's exclusive use.

5.   Nappies, pins and pants (or disposable nappies). Ideally about three dozen if they are towelling. A huge supply if they are disposable.

6.   Zinc and castor oil cream, or Vaseline, to 'waterproof' the bottom.

7.   A 2–3-inch crêpe bandage, and a needle and cotton. This is to secure the cord dressing. The bandage can be obtained on prescription from the chemist if the midwife does not provide it.

8.   Cot or some other sleeping container.

9.   Clothes. The standard layette normally consists of:

3 vests	3 pairs boots and mittens
3 warm gowns	2 shawls
3 jackets or cardigans	2 or 3 baby blankets

The midwife will usually leave a delivery box with the mother from about the thirty-sixth week. In addition to the pack containing the sterilized items necessary for the delivery (bowls, sterile gown, cotton wool, cord clamps and scissors, etc.), it will also contain extra plastic sheets, plastic-backed absorbent pads, extra cotton wool, extra maternity pads, plastic clamps and/or sterilized cord ties, a larger plastic bag for rubbish (to line the cardboard box), a mucus extractor, charts for keeping records of both the mother and baby during and after birth, and a small separate pack containing wool balls and a sterilized foil tray for cleaning the baby's eyes and face. The precise list of contents may vary from region to region. Most community midwives now carry so much equipment with them that it seems unthinkable that years ago they would have walked or cycled to the labouring woman's house. These days, a car seems to be absolutely essential for storage, if not for travel. In addition to the Entonox (gas and air) machine (see pages 106–7), and the bag containing her blood-pressure machine and foetal stethoscope which is brought to antenatal visits at home, the midwife also has a separate delivery bag. A typical list of contents would be:

Clinically clean apron

2 plastic aprons to protect uniform during delivery and when bathing the baby

2 paper hats to keep the midwife's (and if necessary the doctor's) hair out of the way of the actual delivery

Plastic gloves and finger cots for rectal examinations or enema/suppository administration

Sterilized rubber gloves for the delivery and vaginal examinations

Nail brush and paper towels for 'scrubbing up' hands

2 catheters (thin sterilized rubber tubes) for inserting into the bladder of the mother, via the urethra, if she is unable to pass urine

Amnihook for breaking the waters

2 disposable enemas

Disposable razor for perineal shaving, if the mother has to be transferred in labour to a hospital that requires this

Syringes, needles of various sizes and skin sterilizing swabs, all for giving injections

2 mucus extractors

Nitrazene sticks (indicator sticks) for distinguishing amniotic fluid from urine and other liquids

Vaginal examination pack for cleaning the mother's perineum prior to assessing the dilation of the cervix

Disposable speculum for inspecting the cervix

2 ampoules syntometrine and 1 ampoule ergometrine (see page 145)

Ergometrine tablets to be taken orally if necessary, to keep the uterus in a contracted state

Paracetamol tablets to relieve 'after pains' if necessary

1 ampoule Konakion (vitamin K) in injection form for the baby. This is given routinely in some areas to any baby delivered by forceps in the hope that it will reduce the possibility of bruising or bleeding

1 ampoule Coramine, a cardiac stimulant for intramuscular and intravenous use

1 ampoule Xylocaine, a local anaesthetic to be given by injection prior to performing an episiotomy

1 bottle tincture of opium and chloral hydrate. This is a drug given very early on in labour, before the contractions become properly established, to help the mother sleep if she is kept awake at night by irregular tightenings of the uterus

1 bottle magnesium trisilicate, a white liquid tasting like peppermint-flavoured chalk, given during labour to prevent nausea and flatulence, reduce hunger and make the stomach contents alkaline, thereby reducing the dangers associated with inhaling vomit under anaesthetic, should an emergency anaesthetic be needed.

Medicine measure for the preceding two items

Hibitane cream, used for lubrication of the gloved fingers and vagina during assessments of cervical dilation

Olive oil, still used in some areas to clean the vernix off the baby's skin

Silver swaddler, rather like aluminium cooking foil, for wrapping a baby who is born prematurely at home to reduce heat loss during transportation to hospital for special care

Sterzac powder for treating the baby's cord stump

Bottle of antiseptic

Thermometer

Spring balance for weighing the baby

Tape measure for measuring the head circumference and possibly the length of the baby
Sheet of postnatal exercises

All the above can be contained quite adequately in a bag
measuring 18 in by 18 in! The midwife may also bring an
additional bag containing the necessary equipment for giving
intravenous fluids, resuscitating and intubating the baby (intubation is the passage of a small plastic tube down the back
of the baby's throat and down the windpipe to introduce air
or oxygen directly into the lungs), and stitching materials. A
pair of obstetric forceps may be added too, if the GP requests
them.

An outline of the conduct of a home delivery

When the mother feels that she needs the midwife, she will
contact her by phone, either directly or via the midwife's
office or base. Having ascertained that a home visit is necessary, the midwife, possibly with a pupil midwife, will attend
the mother at her home.

The midwife will discuss the events that have taken place
since the phone call, (show? waters broken? frequency,
strength and length of contractions? etc.) and proceed initially
as if it were an antenatal visit – i.e. check the mother's blood
pressure and urine, the baby's position (abdominally) and
heart rate, and in addition the mother's pulse and temperature. She will then examine the mother vaginally or rectally
to determine the state of the cervix and membranes. If the
midwife decides that the mother is in labour, she may trim
the pubic hair (if this seems necessary), and give suppositories
or an enema – again, only if necessary. The mother may take
a bath if she feels she would like one. The GP will be informed
of his patient's condition. If it has not already been prepared,
the bed is made up with newspaper or plastic covering the
mattress, a bottom sheet, a plastic drawsheet and whatever
the mother has provided for use as an upper drawsheet. If the
waters have broken, extra absorbent pads may also be placed

on top. With the newspaper provided the relevant floor area is protected, and the surfaces on which the midwife will work also covered with paper. The midwife then sets out the items necessary for delivery. As with all labours, a careful record of maternal and foetal condition and the progress of labour is kept.

The cot is prepared by wrapping a receiving blanket, towel and baby clothes round a hot water bottle (filled from the kettle) placing this bundle on the bottom cot sheet, then covering it with the remaining cot blankets.

As the second stage approaches the midwife will turn the heating on or up, prepare her equipment and lotions and scrub her hands thoroughly before putting on a gown, hat and gloves. The GP is again informed when delivery is imminent. The mother's perineum is washed with an antiseptic solution and fresh, clean, absorbent material is placed underneath her.

Once the baby is born, his or her eyes may be wiped and his or her nose and mouth cleared of mucus if necessary. The cord is clamped and cut once pulsation has stopped, and the baby is then wrapped in the warmed receiving blanket and given back to the mother. The placenta is delivered and an oxytocic drug may be given (see page 145). The mother's perineum is again cleansed, and vagina and perineum are inspected to see if any lacerations are present which require stitching. Unless the midwife has been specifically instructed in the procedure, the GP will perform the necessary stitching.

The placenta is examined to see whether it is normal and complete, and blood loss is measured.

Postdelivery recordings of temperature, pulse and blood pressure are made, and the state of the mother's uterus is checked. The mother will either be given a wash in bed, to refresh her, or accompanied to the bath or shower. She will be asked to sit on the bedpan or equivalent, so that the amount of urine she passes can be measured. She will then have her vulva and perineum reswabbed and a maternity pad applied. The bed is now changed and the mother is made comfortable. Throughout this a watchful eye has been kept on the baby who is now thoroughly inspected by the midwife and/or the GP for any 'defects'. He or she is weighed in a nappy (like a stork bundle!), all four corners secured and attached to a spring balance. The baby's temperature is recorded and he is then washed or bathed (according to the mother's inclinations), dried and dressed. The cord stump is treated by tying it in three places with sterile string, applying a 'key-hole' dressing and powdering liberally with Sterzac. The 'parcel' of cord and powder is then secured with crêpe bandage and sewn into place. If the baby has not already done so, he will probably now go to the breast for his first feed, under the midwife's supervision if necessary. The equipment is packed up, newspaper collected and all rubbish and placenta are wrapped and taken away to be incinerated, in the cardboard box lined with a plastic rubbish bag. The room is left clean and tidy, and mother left to rest until the return visit two hours later. The District Medical Officer is notified of the birth.

N.B. This account is not intended to be exhaustive, and the reader must also appreciate that considerable variation is likely according to the facilities available to the midwife, and the practices of the area in which she works.

Appendix 3

Active birth

Doctor Michel Odent is the director of a nineteen-bed maternity unit at the Centre Hospitalier General de Pithiviers, France. Pithiviers itself is a small town 60 kilometres south of Paris with a population of about 45,000. The hospital provides maternity care for the local population without selection; mothers with obstetric complications are all admitted. In addition, about 40 per cent of the 900 mothers delivered there each year come from outside the area, sometimes from outside the country. Professional care is provided by Dr Odent (or a colleague) and six midwives. The midwives work in pairs for periods of forty-eight hours which they spend entirely in the unit; they then have four days off duty. Antenatal care is shared between the mother's own family doctor and the maternity unit.

In this unit Dr Odent has been able to put his own philosophy into practice. His philosophy has evolved in part from ideas first launched by the French obstetrician Frederick Leboyer in 1974 in his book *Pour une naissance sans violence* (translated into English as *Birth Without Violence*, Fontana/Collins, 1977). He has also been influenced by the works of Wilhelm Reich (vegetotherapy), Bernard This (a French psychoanalyst) and Madame Marie Louise Aucher, who founded what is now known as 'Psychophonie' in France. This is a means of developing the potential of any human being, and, in connection with birth, is concerned with the effect of the mother's voice on her unborn child. These, and many other topics, are discussed in his two books *Bien Naître* ('Born well'), Editions du Seuil, Paris, 1976, and *Genèse de l'homme écologique: l'instinct retrouvé* ('Genesis of ecological man: the natural instinct rediscovered'), Editions de l'Epi, Paris, 1979. (Neither of these two books are yet available in English translations.)

One of the central beliefs that colours much of the practices at the maternity unit is that the normal physiology of the birth process should not be disturbed, and that the atmosphere of the hospital, the behaviour of the staff, and the environment in which the mother gives birth, should all facilitate the change in level of consciousness in the labouring woman which is seen as an integral part of normal labour.

Dr Odent describes this process as 'regression', during which the mother in labour separates herself from her modern world so that she forgets what is learned or cultural, and instead responds to what is instinctive inside herself, as if listening to an older, more primitive part of her brain. Such regression frees the emotions and releases the body. In this state the mother adopts positions that she finds helpful and is able to relax both sphincter and perineal muscles. He suggests that this altering of the state of consciousness protects the mother against the effects of pain and produces a positive sense of wellbeing. One possible explanation for this is that there is an optimum state of consciousness for the *inhibition* of adrenergic secretions, the hormones such as adrenaline which produce the 'fight or flight' response in humans as well as animals, and the *release* of oxytocin and even perhaps endorphins – the 'endogenous opiates' of the brain.

Accordingly, preparations for birth take the form of weekly group discussions to which the husbands come. These meetings emphasize the excitement, happiness and normality of birth. They include evenings of singing led by Madame Aucher, and discussions with newly delivered parents. Most mothers are admitted in labour since *induction is not practised*. Each mother is given her own bed in a single- or double-bedded room which she keeps throughout her stay. There are few rules, and the mother wears her own nightclothes. The mother is encouraged to stay upright and walk about during the first stage of labour, and as labour advances she makes her way to the delivery suite which includes two conventional labour rooms, which are rarely used except for medical procedures and instrumental (ventouse) deliveries, and a third, 'birth room', the *salle sauvage*. (Caesarean sections are done in the surgical department of the hospital.)

The birth room is predominantly brown, with orange curtains at the windows. There is no clock and a raffia shade covers the light bulb. In one corner of the room there is a large, firm, low-level platform with many brightly coloured cushions, a record player, and a birth chair. Extra heating is always available from a small heater. The lighting in the birth room is subdued to reduce unnecessary sensory stimuli, and the birth attendants recognize the importance of silence and of substituting soothing music for distracting noises. Communication with the mother is also on a 'basic' level, with simple words which spare the intellect, or by touch and gesture. The mother is emotionally supported in labour by as few people as possible, and by people she knows and trusts. The midwife, her husband, her mother – the male doctor, or male observers are excluded as far as possible as the presence of a man is observed to produce a negative effect in some cases.

A small, inflatable pool of warm water is also available for the mother to use as an aid to relaxation. Some mothers find this so helpful that they spend their entire labour in the pool. Although this is not actively encouraged, about eighty babies a year are born while the mother is in the water, and seem to come to no harm.

During the second stage the mother is again encouraged to 'listen' to her own body's needs and adopt positions conducive to her comfort and relaxation. Michel Odent believes that the positions a mother adopts in labour and her state of consciousness are reciprocal, i.e. that the mother needs to be free to find postures which, traditionally, have been used to facilitate altered states of consciousness, such as kneeling on all fours as if praying, and that conversely 'liberating the instinctive brain' increases the capacity to find spontaneously positions which are physiologically effective, for example, the baby's head rotates more easily in the pelvis when the mother is on all fours.

Over the years, the mothers delivering in the unit have been observed to adopt a variety of positions: kneeling, standing, sitting, curled up on the side, crouching, squatting and bending forwards from a standing or kneeling position, as well as a variety of asymmetrical positions, for example, with one leg straight out, or leaning to one side.

At the end of the second stage, when a standing woman experiences a contraction she is normally observed to bend her knees to squat, especially if one or two assistants are supporting her shoulders. This position seems to be the most efficient as it produces the maximum pressure in the pelvis, the greatest increase in the surface areas of the pelvic outlet, the minimum muscular effort and the optimum relaxation of the pelvic muscles. If the mother is giving birth to a baby in the breech position, Dr Odent feels that this position is essential to avoid delay between the delivery of the baby and umbilical cord, and the delivery of the head. During this interval the baby's blood (and therefore oxygen) supply is being reduced as the cord is compressed (at least partially) between the baby's head and the mother's pelvis. The upright position also greatly reduces the need for episiotomy, which is only *7 per cent for the whole unit*. The baby is delivered towards the mother who sits down, or sits back on her heels, takes the child in her arms and puts it to her breast within minutes of its being born. The *cord is not clamped* or cut until the baby is at least five minutes old, and the cord has stopped pulsating, and *no oxytocic agents*, e.g. syntometrine or ergometrine, are given to the mother routinely.

The placenta is delivered by gravity and the mother's own effort, or by gentle cord traction.

The mother is given a bowl of warm water which is placed between her legs. Into this she lowers her baby for a few minutes, washing, observing and talking to him. After this, the baby is dried, wrapped and given to the father while the mother is washed. Then the mother and father walk, carrying their new baby, back to the mother's room.

The whole policy is one of non-intervention and minimum disturbance of the normal physiology. The *mother is given no analgesics* or other drugs in labour and her *membranes are not broken artificially.*

Forceps are not used in the unit. If obstetric assistance is required the mother is either delivered using the ventouse or vacuum extractor, or by Caesarean section.

During the years 1977 and 1978 Dr Odent and his midwives acted chiefly as observers; no directions or instructions were given to the mother which would influence or limit her own inclinations in labour. During this period 1799 babies were delivered, of which 1592 (88.5 per cent) were delivered spontaneously, 58 (3.2 per cent) were delivered by vacuum extraction and 149 (8.3 per cent) by Caesarean section. Over the same period 16 babies died (0.9 per cent), 31 (1.7 per cent) were transferred after birth to specialist units because of major neonatal problems, and 17 (1 per cent) of mothers required manual removal for the delivery of the placenta. Unfortunately, figures such as these can only become significant when compared with those obtained from a unit or hospital which serves a comparable population, and the mothers that have their babies in the Pithiviers hospital may well be unique in terms of the population of which they are a part.

Appendix 4

Coping with perineal stitches

Some practical advice

1. As soon as possible after delivery, the mother should start to move the pelvic floor muscles: she should be persuaded to squeeze the muscles and let go, frequently. She will probably be reluctant to do so at first, because it hurts to start with, but such movements, however slight, help to disperse waste products and reduce swelling, like a soapy sponge being cleansed in the bath water.[1]

2. While passing urine, an attempt should be made to stop and restart the urine stream. This will again probably be very difficult at first, even for a woman who was conscientious about doing pelvic floor exercises antenatally, but with practice the ability will return.

3. While passing urine, she will find that a jug full of warm water poured over the vulva and perineum will help to dilute the urine and prevent stinging of any lacerations of the labia or vagina.

4. It is vital to keep the stitched area clean and dry. In hospital this may be effected by the use of the bidet – at home running water may be used by means of a jug, crouching in the bath with a shower attachment on the taps and the jet

directed onto the perineum, or best of all, (in the absence of a bidet) a shower at the side of the toilet can be used to direct a stream of water at the perineum while the mother sits on the toilet. A useful alternative to all of the above is an empty washing-up liquid bottle which can be filled with lukewarm water and directed at the perineum.

5.   Tissues or soft toilet paper are best used to dry the perineal area. These are gentle and very absorbent, so that the mother will be less inclined to skimp drying because it hurts.

6.   In the early days a clean sanitary pad should be put on each time the mother visits the toilet. She needs to experiment to find the texture and type of pad which suits her best: in general the soft absorbent material of the nondisposable type is more gentle on the stitch line. Pads should be detached front first and removed from behind. Some mothers, who do not find the presence of a sanitary belt round their newly delivered 'waist' too uncomfortable, may find that a pad which is held firmly against the perineum is less likely to rub on their stitches than a disposable type of pad which sticks on the gusset of the pants.

7.   Wiping after evacuation of the bowel should always be done from front to back to avoid contaminating the stitch line.

8.   The exposure of the stitched perineum to the light and heat of an ordinary light bulb (from an anglepoise lamp for greater convenience) may be very soothing. It also dries the area and speeds healing.

9.   The stitched area may be slightly tender even though the skin is healed, so experimentation with positions in lovemaking may be appropriate, to find one which does not put pressure on the scar.

10.   It has recently been found that ultrasound is a very effective method of treating thickened scars which cause pain. A five-minute application, three times a week for six weeks, is a typical treatment scheme. This has been effective even

when the woman has not sought help until fifteen or even forty-eight weeks after episiotomy.[2]

Appendix 5

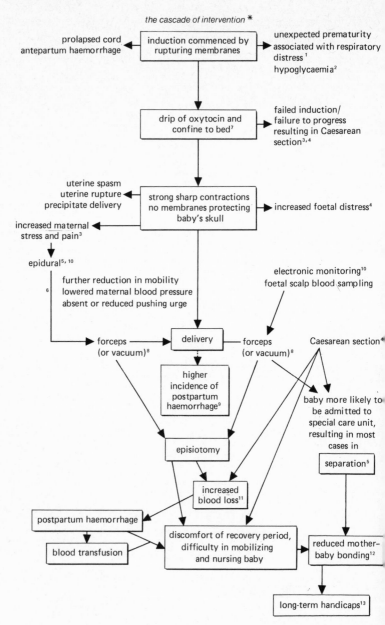

the cascade of intervention *

induction commenced by rupturing membranes
→ prolapsed cord
antepartum haemorrhage
→ unexpected prematurity associated with respiratory distress [1]
hypoglycaemia [2]

drip of oxytocin and confine to bed [7]
→ failed induction/ failure to progress resulting in Caesarean section [3,4]

strong sharp contractions no membranes protecting baby's skull
→ uterine spasm
uterine rupture
precipitate delivery
→ increased foetal distress [4]

increased maternal stress and pain [3]

epidural [5,10]

further reduction in mobility
lowered maternal blood pressure
absent or reduced pushing urge [6]

electronic monitoring [10]
foetal scalp blood sampling

forceps (or vacuum) [8]

delivery

forceps (or vacuum) [8]

Caesarean section *

higher incidence of postpartum haemorrhage [9]

baby more likely to be admitted to special care unit, resulting in most cases in

separation [5]

episiotomy

increased blood loss [11]

postpartum haemorrhage

blood transfusion

discomfort of recovery period, difficulty in mobilizing and nursing baby

reduced mother–baby bonding [12]

long-term handicaps [13]

* Adapted from material supplied by A. H. MacLennan.

References

The evolution of the midwife

1. T. Szasz, *The Manufacture of Madness*, Paladin, 1973.
2. Barbara Ehrenreich and Deirdre English, *Witches, Midwives and Nurses*, Compendium, 1974.
3. F. Mauriceau, *The Diseases of Women with Child and in Childbed*, trans. by Hugh Chamberlen, 3rd edn, London, 1697.

The assumption of pathology

1. *Peel Committee Report*, Standing Maternity and Midwifery Advisory Committee, HMSO, 1970.
2. Marjorie Tew, in S. Kitzinger and J. Davis (eds.), *Place of Birth*, Oxford University Press, 1978, p. 56.
3. J. G. Fryer and J. R. Ashford, *British Journal of Preventative and Social Medicine*, 26, 1972, pp. 1–9.
4. J. R. Ashford, in Kitzinger and Davis, op. cit., p. 33.
5. Marjorie Tew, in Kitzinger and Davis, op. cit., p. 64.
6. G. Chamberlain *et al.*, *British Births 1970*, Heinemann, 1975.
7. *Registrar General's Statistical Review of England and Wales, 1962–73*, HMSO, 1976.
8. G. L. Kloosterman, quoted in Suzanne Arms, *Immaculate Deception*, Houghton Mifflin, Boston, 1975, p. 287.
9. W. O. M. Moore, in Kitzinger and Davis, op. cit., p. 4.

10. K. R. Niswander and M. Gordon, *The Women and Their Pregnancies*, Collaborative Study of the National Institute of Neurological Diseases and Stroke, W. B. Saunders, Philadelphia, 1972, p. 126.

11. G. Ferster and R. J. Pethybridge, *Hospital and Health Services Review*, 1973, pp. 243–7.

12. J. A. Stilwen, *British Medical Journal*, 2, 1979, pp. 257–9.

13. National Perinatal Epidemiology Unit, quoted in the *Guardian*, 20 October 1979, p. 5.

14. Marjorie Tew, 'The safest place of birth – further evidence', *Lancet*, 30 June 1979, pp. 1388–90.

15. M. P. M. Richards, in Kitzinger and Davis, op. cit., p. 72.

16. M. P. M. Richards, 'Obstetricians and the induction of labour in Britain', *Social Science and Medicine*, 9, 1975, pp. 595–602; 'The induction and acceleration of labour: some benefits and complications', *Early Human Development*, 1 (3-A), 1977.

17. M. P. M. Richards, in Kitzinger and Davis, op. cit., p. 78.

18. J. H. E. Carmichael and R. J. Berry, 'Diagnostic X-rays in late pregnancy and in the neonate', *Lancet*, 1, 1976, p. 351.

19. I. Chalmers, 'Evaluation of different approaches to obstetric care', paper presented to a seminar on Human Relations and Obstetric Practice, University of Warwick, October, 1975.

20. H. G. Mahler, *Lancet*, 2, 1 November 1975, pp. 829–33.

21. H. G. Mather *et al.*, 'Myocardial infarction – a comparison between home and hospital care for patients', *British Medical Journal*, 1, 1976, p. 925.

22. K. O'Driscoll *et al.*, 'Selective induction of labour, *British Medical Journal*, 4, 1975, pp. 727–9.

23. A. L. Cochrane, *Effectiveness and Efficiency*, Oxford University Press for the Nuffield Perinatal Hospitals Trust, 1972.

24. D. P. Byar, R. M. Simon, W. T. Friedewald *et al.*, 'Randomized clinical trials', *New England Journal of Medicine*, 295, 1976, p. 74.

25. L. W. Shaw and T. C. Chalmers, 'Ethics in cooperative clinical trials', *Annals of the New York Academy of Science*, 169, 1970, p. 487.

26. W. R. Rosengren and S. De Vault, 'Impact of hospital routines on the management of the different stages of birth', in E. Friedson (ed.), *The Hospital in Modern Society*, Free Press of Glencoe, New York, 1963.

27. G. L. Kloosterman, in Suzanne Arms, op. cit.

28. P. Dunn, 'Obstetric delivery today', *Lancet*, 10 April 1976, pp. 790–93.

29. A. H. MacLennan, 'An audit of obstetric practice in the management of labour', *Australian and New Zealand Journal of Obstetrics and Gynaecology*, 18, 1978, pp. 287–8.

30. A. H. MacLennan, personal communication, 1980 (reproduced by kind permission).

31. D. Riley, 'What do women want? The question of choice in the conduct of labour', in T. Chard and M. Richards (eds.), *Benefits and Hazards of the New Obstetrics*, Heinemann, 1977.

32. E. Shabanah, A. Toth and G. B. Maughan, *American Journal of Obstetrics and Gynaecology*, 89, 1977, p. 841.

33. M. Newton, M. Newton and D. Peeler, 'Effects of disturbance on labour', *American Journal of Obstetrics and Gynaecology*, 101, 1968, pp. 1096–102.

34. E. A. Williams, *Journal of Obstetrics and Gynaecology of the British Empire*, 59, 1952, p. 635.

35. J. Kelly, 'Effect of fear on uterine motility', *American Journal of Obstetrics and Gynaecology*, 83, 1962, pp. 576–81.

36. H. Fox, *Birth and the Family Journal*, 6(3), 1979, p. 162.

37. M. Enkin, *Birth and the Family Journal*, 4(3), 1977, p. 101.

38. M. Richards, 'An evaluation of the risks of hospital delivery', in Kitzinger and Davis, op. cit., p. 71.

39. A. W. Franklin, 'A fresh look at childbirth', *Journal of Maternal and Child Health*, January 1980.

3 The first stage: Alterations of the physiological pattern

1. J. B. De Lee, *Obstetrics for Nurses*, W. B. Saunders, Philadelphia, 1904.

2. M. Myles, *Textbook for Midwives*, 7th edn, Churchill & Livingstone, Edinburgh and London, 1972.

3. M. Romney, 'Predelivery shaving: an unjustified assault?', *Journal of Obstetrics and Gynaecology*, 1(1), 1980, pp. 33–5.

4. T. Denman, *An Introduction to the Practice of Midwifery*, E. Bliss & E. White, New York, 1821.

5. F. Churchill, *On the Theory and Practice of Midwifery*, 3rd edn, Lea, Philadelphia, 1848.

6. G. S. Bedford, *The Principles and Practice of Obstetrics*, 4th edn, William Wood & Co., New York, 1868.

7. S. P. Warren, 'Technique of labour in private practice', *Amer-*

ican Journal of Obstetrics and Diseases of Woman and Child, 45, 1902, p. 26.

8. J. W. Williams, *Obstetrics: A Textbook for the Use of Students and Practitioners*, 1st–5th edns, Appleton, New York.

9. R. A. Johnston and R. S. Sidall, 'Is the usual method of preparing patients for delivery beneficial or necessary?', *American Journal of Obstetrics and Gynaecology*, 4, 1922, pp. 645–50.

10. H. Lankford, *American Journal of Obstetrics and Gynaecology*, 2, 1921, pp. 176–8.

11. R. Burchell, 'Predelivery removal of pubic hair', *Obstetrics and Gynaecology*, 24, 1964, pp. 272–3.

12. H. Kantor *et al.*, 'Value of shaving the pudendal-perineal area in delivery preparation', *Obstetrics and Gynaecology*, 25, 1965, pp. 509–12.

13. P. Lomas, in S. Kitzinger and J. Davis (eds.), *Place of Birth*, Oxford University Press, 1978.

14. F. Mauriceau, *Observations sur la grossesse et l'accouchement*, 1668; translated by Hugh Chamberlen as *The Accomplisht Midwife*, 1673 and (3rd edn.) *The Diseases of Women with Child and in Childbed*, 1697.

15. S. Merriman, *A Synopsis of the Various Kinds of Difficult Parturition, with Practical Remarks on the Management of Labours*, Stonehouse, Philadelphia, 1816.

16. G. J. Engelmann, *Labour Among Primitive Peoples*, St Louis, 1882.

17. W. T. Lusk, *The Science and Art of Midwifery*, D. Appleton, New York, 1894.

18. W. Smellie, in A. H. McClintoch (ed.), *Treatise on the Theory and Practice of Midwifery*, London, 1876.

19. D. B. Scott and M. G. Kerr, *Journal of Obstetrics and Gynaecology of the British Commonwealth*, 7, 1963, p. 1044.

20. C. J. Mendez-Bauer, *Journal of Perinatal Medicine*, 3, 1975, p. 89.

21. R. Schwarcz, A. G. Diaz, R. Fescina, R. Caldeyro-Barcia, *Latin American Collaborative Study on Maternal Posture in Labour*, 1977; reported in *Birth and the Family Journal*, 6(1), 1979.

22. R. Schwarcz *et al.*, *Proceedings of the VII World Congress of Gynaecology and Obstetrics*, Excerpta Medica, North Holland, 1976, pp. 377–91.

23. P. Dunn, 'Obstetric delivery today', *Lancet*, 10 April 1976, pp. 790–93.

24. Margaret Mead, in S. A. Richardson and A. F. Guttmacher

(eds.), *Childbearing: Its Social and Psychological Aspects*, Williams & Wilkins, Baltimore, 1967, p. 201.

25. Margaret Mead, *Male and Female: A Study of the Sexes in a Changing World*, Morrow, New York, 1946.

26. E. E. Phillip, *Obstetrics and Gynaecology Combined for Students*, H. K. Lewis, 1962.

27. D. Llewellyn-Jones, *Fundamentals of Obstetrics and Gynaecology*, Faber & Faber, 1969.

28. M. Myles, *Textbook for Midwives*, Churchill Livingstone, Edinburgh, 1972.

4 The first stage: The active management of labour

1. T. Chard, 'The physiology of labour and its initiation', in T. Chard and M. Richards (eds.), *Benefits and Hazards of the New Obstetrics*, Heinemann, 1977.

2. Garvey, Govan, Hodge and Callander, *Obstetrics Illustrated*, 2nd edn, Churchill Livingstone, Edinburgh, 1974, p. 458.

3. W. Patterson, 'Amniotomy, with or without simultaneous oxytocin infusion', *Journal of Obstetrics and Gynaecology of the British Commonwealth*, 78, 1971, pp. 310–16.

4. P. Howie, 'Induction of labour', in Chard and Richards, op. cit.

5. Setna *et al.*, *Journal of Obstetrics and Gynaecology of the British Commonwealth*, 74, 1967, p. 262.

6. A. C. Turnbull and A. M. B. Anderson, *Journal of Obstetrics and Gynaecology of the British Commonwealth*, 75, 1968, p. 32.

7. W. P. Bradford and G. Gordon, *Journal of Obstetrics and Gynaecology of the British Commonwealth*, 75, 1968, p. 698.

8. M. A. Garud and S. C. Simmons, *Journal of Obstetrics and Gynaecology of the British Commonwealth*, 75, 1968, p. 702.

9. M. E. Pawson and S. C. Simmons, *British Medical Journal*, 3, 1970, p. 191.

10. P. J. Steer *et al.*, 'Uterine activity in induced labour', *British Journal of Obstetrics and Gynaecology*, 83, 1975, pp. 454–9.

11. N. G. Caseby, 'Epidural analgesia for the surgical induction of labour', *British Journal of Anaesthesia*, 46, 1974, pp. 747–51.

12. D. Llewellyn-Jones, *Fundamentals of Obstetrics and Gynaecology*, vol. 1: *Obstetrics*, Faber & Faber, 1969, p. 335.

13. S. M. M. Karim *et al.*, 'Response of the pregnant human uterus

to prostaglandin F_2X induction of labour', *British Medical Journal*, 4, 1968, pp. 621–3.

14. I. Z. Mackenzie and M. P. Embrey, *British Medical Journal*, 2, 1977, p. 1381.

15. A. A. Calder and M. P. Embrey, 'Induction of labour', in R. Beard, M. Brudenell, P. Dunn and D. Fairweather (eds.), *The Management of Labour*, Proceedings of the Third Study Group of the Royal College of Obstetricians and Gynaecologists, London, 1975, p. 62.

16. D. R. Bromham and R. S. Anderson, 'Uterine scar rupture in labour induced with vaginal prostaglandin E_2', *Lancet*, 30 August 1980, p. 485.

17. A. P. Gordon-Wright and M. G. Elder, *British Journal of Obstetrics and Gynaecology*, 86, 1979, pp. 32–6.

18. J. F. Miller, G. A. Welply and M. Elstein, *British Medical Journal*, 1, 1975, p. 14.

19. P. Yudkin, A. M. Frumar, A. M. B. Anderson and A. C. Turnbull, 'A retrospective study of induction of labour', *British Journal of Obstetrics and Gynaecology*, 86(4), 1979, pp. 257–65.

20. I. Chalmers, 'Evaluation of different approaches to obstetric care', paper presented to a seminar on Human Relations and Obstetric Practice, University of Warwick, October 1975.

21. J. Bonnar, 'Induction and acceleration of labour in modern obstetric practice', paper presented at a study group on Problems in Obstetrics by the Medical Information Unit of the Spastics Society, 1975.

22. H. Arthure *et al.*, 'Report on confidential inquiries into maternal deaths. Tunbridge Wells, April 1975', in *England and Wales 1970–72*, DHSS report on Health and Social Subjects, no. 11, HMSO, 1975.

23. K. O'Driscoll, 'An obstetrician's view of pain', *British Journal of Anaesthesia*, 47, 1975, pp. 1053–9.

24. I. J. Hoult, A. H. MacLennan and L. E. S. Carrie, *British Medical Journal*, 1, 1977, p. 14.

25. W. A. Liston and A. J. Campbell, *British Medical Journal*, 3, 1974, p. 606.

26. P. R. S. Brinsden and A. D. Clarke, 'Postpartum haemorrhage after induced and spontaneous labours', *British Medical Journal*, 2, 1978, pp. 855–6.

27. M. E. Pawson and S. C. Simmons, *British Medical Journal*, 3, 1970, p. 191.

28. K. Hartman, paper given to the GP Obstetric Unit meeting on the MM2, John Radcliffe Hospital, Oxford, March 1979.

29. I. Chalmers *et al.*, 'Obstetric practice and outcome of pregnancy in Cardiff residents, 1965–73', *British Medical Journal*, 1, 1976, pp. 735–8.

30. A. Ghosh, 'Oxytocic agents and neonatal morbidity', *Lancet*, 1, 1975, p. 453.

31. M. Richards, 'Induction and acceleration of labour – some benefits and complications', *Early Human Development*, 1, 1977, pp. 3–17.

32. R. Caldeyro-Barcia, quoted in Suzanne Arms, *Immaculate Deception*, Houghton Mifflin, Boston, 1975.

33. W. A. Bowes, Y. Brackbill, E. Conway and A. Steinschneider (eds.), 'The effects of obstetric induction on foetus and infant', *Monographs of the Society for Research in Child Development*, no. 4, 1970, p. 137.

34. M. K. Aleksandrowicz, 'The effects of pain-relieving drugs administered during labour and delivery on the behaviour of the newborn: a review', *Merrill-Palmer Quarterly*, 20, 1974, pp. 121–41.

35. J. W. Scanlon, 'Obstetric anaesthesia as a neonatal risk factor in normal labour and delivery', *Clinics in Perinatology*, 1, 1974, pp. 465–82.

36. J. S. McDonald, L. L. Bjorkman and E. C. Reed, 'Epidural anaesthesia for obstetrics', *American Journal of Obstetrics and Gynaecology*, 120, 1974, p. 1055.

37. M. Richards, 'An examination of the risks of hospital delivery', in S. Kitzinger and J. Davis (eds.), *Place of Birth*, Oxford University Press, 1978.

38. I. Chalmers, H. Campbell and A. C. Turnbull, 'Use of oxytocin and incidence of neonatal jaundice', *British Medical Journal*, 1, 1975, pp. 116–18.

39. H. Campbell *et al.*, 'Increased frequency of neonatal jaundice in a maternity hospital', *British Medical Journal*, 3, 1975, pp. 548–52.

40. E. A. Friedman and M. R. Sachtleben, 'Neonatal jaundice in association with oxytocin stimulation of labour and operative delivery', *British Medical Journal*, 1, 1976, pp. 198–9.

41. D. Llewellyn-Jones, *Fundamentals of Obstetrics and Gynaecology*, vol. 1: *Obstetrics*, part 3, Faber & Faber, 1969.

42. E. G. Knox, 'Control of haemolytic disease in the newborn',

British Journal of Preventative and Social Medicine, 30, 1976, pp. 163–9.

43. E. Alberman, 'Facts and figures', in Chard and Richards, op. cit.

44. J. Leeson and A. Smith, *British Medical Journal*, correspondence, 12 March 1977.

45. K. O'Driscoll, C. J. Carroll and M. Coughlan, 'Selective induction of labour', *British Medical Journal*, 4, 1975, pp. 727–9.

46. M. B. McNay, G. W. McIlwaine, P. W. Howie and M. C. MacNaughton, *British Medical Journal*, 1, 5 February 1977, p. 347.

47. I. Chalmers, R. G. Newcombe and H. Campbell, *British Medical Journal*, correspondence, 12 March 1977, p. 707.

48. D. Meager and K. O'Driscoll, *British Medical Journal*, correspondence, 12 March 1977.

49. I. Chalmers, 'Implications of the current debate on obstetric practice', in Kitzinger and Davis, op. cit.

50. I. Chalmers, J. G. Lawson and A. C. Turnbull, 'An evaluation of different approaches to obstetric care', *British Journal of Obstetrics and Gynaecology*, 83, 1976, p. 921.

51. M. Hall *et al.*, 'Is routine antenatal care worthwhile?', *Lancet*, 12 July 1980, pp. 78–80.

52. R. W. Beard, 'Prevention of handicap through antenatal care', in A. C. Turnbull and F. P. Woodford (eds.), *Excerpta Medica*, North Holland, 1976, p. 169.

53. J. F. Pearson and J. B. Weaver, 'Foetal activity and foetal wellbeing: an evaluation', *British Medical Journal*, 1, 1976, pp. 1305–7.

54. N. R. Bulter and D. G. Bonham, *Perinatal Mortality*, Livingstone, Edinburgh, 1963, pp. 113 and 89.

55. J. Schneider *et al.*, 'Screening for foetal and neonatal risk in postdate pregnancy', *American Journal of Obstetrics and Gynaecology*, 131(5), 1978, p. 473.

56. R. Homburg *et al.*, 'Detection of foetal risk in postmaturity', *British Journal of Obstetrics and Gynaecology*, 86, 1979, pp. 759–64.

57. A. MacLennan, 'An audit of obstetric practice in the management of labour', *Australian and New Zealand Journal of Obstetrics and Gynaecology*, 18(4), 1978, pp. 287–8.

58. I. Chalmers and M. Richards, 'Intervention and causal inference in obstetric practice', in Chard and Richards, op. cit.

59. D. Llewellyn-Jones, op. cit., ch. 45.

60. J. Sturrock and R. Brown, in Llewellyn-Jones, op. cit.

61. K. O'Driscoll, 'An obstetrician's view of pain', *British Journal of Anaesthesia*, 47, 1975, p. 1053.

62. R. Schwarcz *et al.*, 'Third progress report on the Latin American collaborative study of the effects of late rupture of the membranes on labour and the neonate', submitted to the Director of the Pan-American Health Organization (PAHO) and the participating groups, Latin American Center of Perinatology and Human Development, Montevideo, 1974; reported in L. Gluck (ed.), *Modern Perinatal Medicine*, Year Book Medical Publishers, Chicago, December 1974, p. 435.

63. R. Schwarcz *et al.*, 'Foetal heart-rate patterns in labour with intact and ruptured membranes', *Journal of Perinatal Medicine*, 1, 1973, p. 153.

64. R. Caldeyro-Barcia, 'Possible iatrogenic effects of rupture of the membranes during foetal monitoring', in J. W. Dudenhausen and E. Saling (eds.), *Perinatale Medizin*, vol. 4, Deutscher Kongress für perinatale Medizin, Georg Thieme Verlag, Stuttgart, 1973, p. 5.

65. R. Caldeyro-Barcia *et al.*, 'Foetal monitoring in labour', in H. M. Wallace, E. M. Gold and E. F. Lis (eds.), *Maternal and Child Health Practices: Problems, Resources and Methods of Delivery*, Chas. C. Thomas, Springfield, Ill., 1973.

66. R. Schwarcz *et al.*; see reference 62 above, p. 432.

67. R. Schwarcz, A. G. Diaz, R. Fescina and R. Caldeyro-Barcia, Latin American Collaborative Study on Maternal Position in Labour; reported in *Birth and the Family Journal*, 6(1), 1979.

68. R. Schwarcz *et al.*; see reference 62 above, p. 433.

69. R. Caldeyro-Barcia, *Birth and the Family Journal*, 2(2), 1975.

70. R. Caldeyro-Barcia, Conference of the American Foundation for Maternal and Child Health, March 1974; reported in Suzanne Arms, *Immaculate Deception*, Houghton Mifflin, Boston, 1975.

71. L. Lindgren, 'The causes of foetal head moulding in labour', *Acta Obstetrica et Gynaecologica Scandanavica*, 38, 1959, p. 211.

72. R. Schwarcz *et al.*, 'Pressure exerted by uterine contractions on the head of the human foetus in labour', in R. Caldeyro-Barcia (moderator), *Perinatal Factors Affecting Human Development*, Pan-American Health Organization, Washington, DC, 1969.

73. E. Holland, 'Cranial stress in the foetus during labour and the

effects of excessive stress on the intercranial contents, with an analysis of 81 cases of torn tenterium cerebrelli and subdural cerebral haemorrhage', *Journal of Obstetrics and Gynaecology of the British Empire*, 29, 1922, p. 549.

74. J. Frederic and N. R. Butler, 'Certain causes of neonatal death: cerebral birth trauma', *Biology of the Neonate*, 18, 1971, p. 321.

75. P. F. Muller *et al.*, 'Perinatal factors and their relationship to mental retardation and other parameters of development', *American Journal of Obstetrics and Gynaecology*, 109, 1971, p. 1205.

76. R. Schwarcz *et al.*; see reference 62 above, p. 437.

77. R. Schwarcz *et al.*; see reference 62 above, p. 439.

78. P. Schwartz, 'Birth injuries in the newborn', *Morphology, Parthogenesis, Clinical Pathology and Prevention*, Hofner Publishing Co. Inc., New York, 1961.

79. G. Aramburu, O. Althabe and R. Caldeyro-Barcia, 'Obstetrical factors influencing compression of the foetal head and the incidence of dips I in foetal heart rate', in C. R. Angle and E. A. Bering (eds.), *Physiological Trauma as an Etiological Agent in Mental Retardation*, US Department of Health, Education and Welfare, NINDS, Bethesda, Md, 1970.

80. O. Althabe *et al.*, 'Influence of the rupture of the membranes on compression of the foetal head in labour', in R. Caldeyro-Barcia (moderator), *Perinatal Factors Affecting Human Development*, Pan-American Health Organization, Washington, DC, 1969.

81. R. Schwarcz *et al.*; see reference 62 above, p. 442.

82. K. R. Niswander and M. Gordon, *The Women and Their Pregnancies*, Collaborative Study of the National Institute of Neurological Diseases and Strokes, W. B. Saunders, Philadelphia, 1972.

83. E. J. Quilligan, 'The obstetric intensive-care unit', *Hospital Practice*, 7, 1972, pp. 61–9.

84. H. A. Gabert and M. A. Stenchever, 'Continuous electronic monitoring of foetal heart rate during labour', *American Journal of Obstetrics and Gynaecology*, 115, 1973, pp. 919–23.

85. R. W. Beard *et al.*, 'The effects of routine ultrapartum monitoring on clinical practice', *Gynaecology and Obstetrics*, 3, 1977, pp. 14–21.

86. I. M. Kelso *et al.*, 'An assessment of continuous foetal heart-

rate monitoring in labour', *American Journal of Obstetrics and Gynaecology*, 131, 1978, pp. 526–32.

87. J. Wennberg, Presentation to the arrival meeting of the American Public Health Association, Los Angeles, October 1978.

88. T. Chard, 'The foetus at risk', *Lancet*, 2, 1974, pp. 880–83.

89. R. L. Caldeyro-Barcia, *Birth and the Family Journal*, 2, (1), 1975, p. 38.

90. M. Balfour *et al.*, 'Complications of foetal blood sampling', *American Journal of Obstetrics and Gynaecology*, 107, 1970, pp. 288–94.

91. H. M. Feder *et al.*, 'Scalp abcess secondary to foetal scalp electrode', *Journal of Paediatrics*, 89, 1976, pp. 808–9.

92. F. J. Plavidal and A. Weroh, 'Foetal scalp abcess secondary to intrauterine monitoring', *American Journal of Obstetrics and Gynaecology*, 125, 1976, pp. 65–70.

93. D. M. Okada *et al.*, 'Neonatal scalp abcesses and foetal monitory factors associated with infection', *American Journal of Obstetrics and Gynaecology*, 129, 1977, pp. 185–9.

94. M. Atlas and D. Serr, 'Hazards of foetal scalp electrodes', *Lancet*, 1, 20 March 1976, p. 648.

95. G. Thomas and R. J. Blacknell, *American Journal of Obstetrics and Gynaecology*, 123, 1973, p. 2118.

96. R. C. Goodlin and J. R. Harrod, *Lancet*, 1, 1973, p. 559.

97. D. F. Tuberville *et al.*, *American Journal of Obstetrics and Gynaecology*, 122, 1975, p. 630.

98. C. B. Gassner and W. J. Ledger, 'The relationship of hospital-acquired maternal infection to invasion intrapartum monitoring techniques', *American Journal of Obstetrics and Gynaecology*, 52, 1978, pp. 193–7.

99. D. Hagen, 'Maternal febrile morbidity associated with foetal monitoring and Caesarean section', *Obstetrics and Gynaecology*, 46, 1975, pp. 260–62.

100. R. H. Paul and E. Mon, 'Clinical foetal monitoring versus effect on perinatal outcome', *American Journal of Obstetrics and Gynaecology*, 118, 1974, pp. 529–33.

101. E. J. Quilligan and R. H. Paul, 'Foetal monitoring – is it worth it?', *Obstetrics and Gynaecology*, 45, 1975, pp. 96–100.

102. A. D. Haverkamp *et al.*, 'The evaluation of continuous foetal heart-rate monitoring in high risk pregnancy', *American Journal of Obstetrics and Gynaecology*, 125, 1976, pp. 310–17.

103. A. D. Haverkamp *et al.*, 'A controlled trial of the differential

effects of intrapartum foetal monitoring', *American Journal of Obstetrics and Gynaecology*, 134, 1979, pp. 399–408.

104. Renou *et al.*, 'Controlled trial of foetal intensive care', *American Journal of Obstetrics and Gynaecology*, 126, 1976, pp. 470–76.

105. D. Banta and S. Thacker, *Birth and the Family Journal*, 6(4), 1979.

106. H. L. Minkoff and R. H. Schwarcz, 'The rising Caesarean-section rate – can it be safely reversed?', *Obstetrics and Gynaecology*, 56, 1980, pp. 135–43.

107. J. R. Evrad and E. M. Gold, 'Caesarean section and maternal mortality in Rhode Island – incidence and risk factors 1965–1975', *Obstetrics and Gynaecology*, 50, 1977, pp. 594–7.

108. H. Arthure *et al.*, *Report on Confidential Inquiries into Maternal Deaths in England and Wales in 1970–72*, Reports of the Health Society, Subject No. 11, HMSO, 1975.

5 The first stage: Pain in labour

1. C. S. McCammon, 'Study of 475 pregnancies in American Indian women', *American Journal of Obstetrics and Gynaecology*, 61, 1951, pp. 1159–66.

2. M. Richards, talk given to the Oxford Postnatal Support Group, 1977.

3. P. Dunn, 'Obstetric delivery today', *Lancet*, April 1976, pp. 790–93.

4. A. Rich, *Of Woman Born*, Virago, 1977, p. 182.

5. H. C. Hutchinson and A. Vasicka, 'Uterine contractility in a paraplegic patient – report of a case', *Obstetrics and Gynaecology*, 20(5), 1963, p. 675.

6. G. Dick Read, *Childbirth Without Fear*, Pan Books, 1968, pp. 62–4.

7. T. Lewis, *Archives of Internal Medicine*, 10(9), May 1932, p. 713.

8. C. Naaktgeboren, quoted in Suzanne Arms, *Immaculate Deception*, Houghton Mifflin, Boston, 1975, pp. 130–32.

9. Doris Haire, *Cultural Warping of Childbirth*, International Childbirth Educational Association, 1972, p. 18.

10. W. A. Brown *et al.*, 'The relationship of antenatal and perinatal psychologic variables to the use of drugs in labour', *Psychosomatic Medicine*, 34, 1972, pp. 119–27.

11. Suzanne Arms, *Immaculate Deception*, Houghton Mifflin, Boston, 1975, p. 126.

12. M. Shearer, paper presented at the Congress of Psychosomatic Obstetrics and Gynaecology, Tel Aviv, 31 October 1974.

13. Doris Haire, op. cit., p. 10.

14. Y. Brackbill, *Birth and the Family Journal*, 5(2), 1978, p. 56.

15. L. Mackenzie, 'Malpractice hazards in obstetrics and gynaecology', *New York State Journal of Medicine*, 1 August 1971, pp. 1877–9.

16. J. Crossland, *Lewis's Pharmacology*, 4th edn, E. and S. Livingstone, Edinburgh, 1970, p. 599.

17. A. R. Petrie *et al.*, 'The effect of drugs on uterine activity', *Obstetrics and Gynaecology*, 48, 1976, pp. 431–5.

18. M. Richards, talk given to the Oxford Postnatal Support Group, 1977.

19. A. M. Grant *et al.*, *Journal of Obstetrics and Gynaecology of the British Commonwealth*, 77, 1970, pp. 824–9.

20. A. Holdcroft and M. Morgan, *Journal of Obstetrics and Gynaecology of the British Commonwealth*, 81, 1974, pp. 603–7.

21. R. E. Kron *et al.*, 'Newborn sucking behaviour affected by obstetric sedation', *Paediatrics*, 37, 1966, p. 1012.

22. J. Dunn and M. P. M. Richards, 'Observations on the developing relationship between mother and baby in the neonatal period', in H. R. Schaffer (ed.), *Studies in Mother–Infant Interaction*, Academic Press, 1977.

23. Y. Brackbill *et al.*, 'Obstetric premedication and infant outcome', *American Journal of Obstetrics and Gynaecology*, 118, 1974, pp. 377–84.

24. W. A. Bowes, Y. Brackbill, E. Conway and A. Steinschreider (eds.), 'The effects of obstetrical medication on foetus and infant', *Monographs of the Society for Research in Child Development*, no. 4, 1970, p. 137.

25. M. I. Hogg *et al.*, 'Urinary excretion of pethedine and norpethedine in the newborn', *British Journal of Anaesthesia*, 49, 1976, pp. 891–9.

26. M. K. Aleksandrowicz, 'The effects of pain-relieving drugs administered in labour and delivery on the behaviour of the newborn: a review', *Merrill-Palmer Quarterly*, 20, 1974, pp. 121–41.

27. M. Richards, 'An examination of the risks of hospital delivery',

in S. Kitzinger and J. Davis (eds.), *Place of Birth*, Oxford University Press, 1976, p. 75.

28. K. A. M. Schott and A. Herz, *European Journal of Pharmacology*, 12, 1970, pp. 53–64.

29. D. Campbell, A. H. B. Mason and W. Norris, *British Journal of Anaesthesia*, 36, 1965, p. 199.

30. M. Richards, 'The one-day-old deprived child', *New Scientist*, 28 March 1974, p. 280.

31. T. N. Evans *et al.*, *British Medical Journal*, 2, 1974, pp. 589–91.

32. M. Rosen, in T. Chard and M. Richards (eds.), *Benefits and Hazards of the New Obstetrics*, Heinemann, 1977, p. 103.

33. A. K. Brown, *Paediatrica*, 53, May 1974, p. 816.

34. M. Rosen, *British Medical Journal*, 3, 1969, pp. 263–7.

35. M. Rosen, 'Survey of current methods of pain relief in labour', in R. Beard, M. Bradwell, P. Dunn and D. Fairweather (eds.), *The Management of Labour*, Proceedings of the Third Study Group of the Royal College of Obstetricians and Gynaecologists, London 1975, pp. 140–48.

36. V. Weiss and G. de Carlini, *Experientia*, 31, 1975, pp. 339–41.

37. M. Rosen, in Chard and Richards, op. cit., p. 109.

38. A. Vasicky, 'Foetal bradycardia after paracervical block', *American Journal of Obstetrics and Gynaecology*, 38, 1971, pp. 500–512.

39. J. Rosefsky and M. Petersiel, 'Perinatal deaths associated with mepivocaine paracervical block anaesthesia in labour', *New England Journal of Medicine*, 278, 1968, pp. 530–33.

40. W. Johnson, 'Regionals can prolong labour', *Medical World News*, 15 October 1971.

41. M. Rosen, in Chard and Richards, op. cit., p. 107.

42. I. J. Hoult, A. H. MacLennan and L. E. S. Carrie, *British Medical Journal*, 1, 1977, pp. 14–16.

43. J. S. McDonald, L. L. Bjorkman and E. C. Reed, 'Epidural analgesia for obstetrics', *American Journal of Obstetrics and Gynaecology*, 120, 1974, p. 1055.

44. B. S. Schifrin, *Journal of Obstetrics and Gynaecology of the British Commonwealth*, 79, 1972, pp. 332–9.

45. G. Thomas, *British Journal of Obstetrics and Gynaecology*, 82, 1975, p. 121.

46. M. Finster and B. S. Bergersen, *Birth and the Family Journal*, 5(2), 1978, p. 77.

47. M. Rosen, in Chard and Richards, op. cit., p. 112.

5 The second stage

1. W. P. Dewees, *System of Midwifery*, quoted by R. Caldeyro-Barcia, *Birth and the Family Journal*, 6(1), 1979, p. 7.

2. R. Caldeyro-Barcia, ibid., p. 10.

3. P. Dunn, 'Obstetric delivery today', *Lancet*, 10 April 1976, pp. 790–93.

4. F. Howard, 'Delivery in the physiologic position', *Obstetrics and Gynaecology*, 11(3), 1958.

5. F. Naroll *et al.*, 'Position of women in childbirth', *American Journal of Obstetrics and Gynaecology*, 82, 1961, pp. 943–54.

6. Human Relations Area Files, *Function and Scope of the Human Relations Area Files*, New Haven, 1954.

7. Human Relations Area Files, *Current Anthropology*, 1, 1960, p. 256.

8. M. Newton, 'The effects of position on the course of the second stage of labour', *Surgical Forum*, 7, 1957, p. 517.

9. N. Newton and M. Newton, 'The propped position for the second stage of labour', *Obstetrics and Gynaecology*, 15(1), 1960).

10. I. J. Hoult, A. H. MacLennan and L. E. S. Carrie, *British Medical Journal*, 1, 1977, pp. 14–16.

11. C. Mendez-Bauer, *Journal of Perinatal Medicine*, 3, 1975, p. 89.

12. F. Howard, 'The application of certain principles of physics to the physiology of delivery', *Western Journal of Surgery*, 62, 1954, p. 607.

13. A. Blankfield, 'The optimum position for childbirth', *Medical Journal of Australia*, 16 October 1965, pp. 666–8.

14. W. F. Mengert and D. P. Murphy, 'Intra-abdominal pressure created by voluntary muscular effort – relation to posture in labour', *Surgery, Gynaecology and Obstetrics*, 57, 1933, pp. 745–51.

15. Doris Haire, *Cultural Warping of Childbirth*, International Childbirth Educational Association, 1972.

16. M. Botha, 'The management of the umbilical cord in labour', *South African Journal of Obstetrics and Gynaecology*, 6(2), 1968, pp. 30–33.

17. A. Beer, 'Foetal erythrocytes in the maternal circulation of 155 Rhesus-negative women', *Obstetrics and Gynaecology*, 34, 1969, pp. 143–50.

18. K. O. Vaughan, *Safe Childbirth: The Three Essentials*, Ballière, Tindall & Cox, 1937.
19. J. G. B. Russell, *Journal of Obstetrics and Gynaecology of the British Commonwealth*, 76, 1969, p. 817.
20. M. Goldman *et al.*, 'Mechanical interaction between the diaphragm and rib cage', *Journal of Applied Physiology*, 35, 1973, p. 197.
21. C. Benyon, 'The normal second stage of labour', *Journal of Obstetrics and Gynaecology of the British Empire*, 64(6), 1957, pp. 185–20.
22. Suzanne Arms, *Immaculate Deception*, Houghton Mifflin, Boston, 1975, p. 143.
23. E. Noble, 'Kaleidoscope of childbearing: preparation, birth and nurturing', paper presented to the Tenth Biennial Convention of the International Childbirth Educational Association, Kansas City, 1978.
24. A. Blankfield, 'The optimum position for childbirth', *Medical Journal of Australia*, 16 October 1965, pp. 666–8.
25. J. V. Basmajian, *Muscles Alive: Their Function Revealed by Electromyography*, 3rd edn, Williams & Wilkins, Baltimore, 1974.
26. E. Agostini *et al.*, 'Electromyography of the diaphragm in man and transdiaphragmatic pressure', *Journal of Applied Physiology*, 15, 1960, pp. 1093–7.
27. M. Moore, 'The conduct of the second stage', in T. Chard and M. Richards (eds.), *Benefits and Hazards of the New Obstetrics*, Heinemann, 1977.
28. R. Caldeyro-Barcia, *Birth and the Family Journal*, 6(1), 1979 pp. 17–21.
29. J. B. De Lee, *The Principles and Practice of Obstetrics*, W. B Saunders, Philadelphia, 1913.
30. T. N. A. Jeffcoate, *British Medical Journal*, 1, 1950, p. 1361.
31. M. Goldman *et al.*, 'Mechanical interaction between the diaphragm and the rib cage', *Journal of Applied Physiology*, 35 1973, p. 197.
32. V. Derbes and A. Kerr, 'Physiological mechanisms', *Cough Syncope*, C. Thomas, 1955.
33. W. R. Cohen, *Obstetrics and Gynaecology*, 49, 1977, pp. 266–9
34. M. L. Brandt, *American Journal of Obstetrics and Gynaecology* 23, 1933, pp. 662–7.

5. M. Myles, *Textbook for Midwives*, Churchill Livingstone, 1972, p. 297.

6. J. Davis, *American Journal of Surgery*, 48, 1940, p. 154.

7. J. R. Fleigner, *Medical Journal of Australia*, 26 August 1978, p. 193.

8. M. M. Pennoyer, *Journal of Paediatrics*, 49, 1956, p. 49.

9. F. K. Graham et al., *Journal of Paediatrics*, 50, 1957, p. 557; B. M. Caldwell, F. K. Graham, M. M. Pennoyer, *Journal of Paediatrics*, 50, 1957, p. 434.

0. N. Cooperman, F. Robovits and F. Hesser, *American Journal of Obstetrics and Gynaecology*, 81(2), 1961, pp. 385–92.

1. I. J. Hoult, A. H. MacLennan and L. E. S. Carrie, *British Medical Journal*, 1, 1977, pp. 14–16.

2. Margaret Mead, in S. A. Richardson and A. F. Guttmacher (eds.), *Childbearing: Its Social and Psychological Aspects*, Williams & Wilkins, Baltimore, 1967, p. 144.

3. J. Burns, *The Principles of Midwifery: Including the Diseases of Women and Children*, Clafton & Van Norden, New York, 1831.

4. S. Merriman, *A Synopsis of the Various Kinds of Difficult Parturition, with Practical Remarks on the Management of Labours*, Stonehouse, Philadelphia, 1816.

5. F. B. Nugent, *American Journal of Obstetrics and Gynaecology*, 30, 1935, pp. 249–56.

6. J. Wilmott, 'Too many episiotomies', *Midwives Chronicle and Nursing Notes*, February 1980, p. 36.

7. L. Mehl et al., 'Home v. hospital delivery: comparisons of matched populations', paper presented at the annual meeting of the American Public Health Association, Miami Beach, Florida, 20 October 1976.

8. I. Chalmers et al., *British Medical Journal*, 1, 1976, pp. 735–8.

9. P. Huntingford, 'Obstetric practice: past, present and future', in S. Kitzinger and J. A. Davis (eds.), *Place of Birth*, Oxford University Press, 1978, pp. 229–50.

0. Personal communication.

1. L. Mehl, G. Peterson and C. Brandsel, 'Episiotomy: facts, fictions, figures and alternatives', in D. and L. Stuart (eds.), *Compulsory Hospitalization or Freedom of Choice in Childbirth?*, NAPSAC Publications, 1979, ch. 15.

2. N. Butler, 'National long-term study of perinatal hazards', paper presented to the Sixth World Conference, Federation of International Gynaecology and Obstetrics, 1970.

53. M. Newton, L. Mosey, G. E. Egli, W. B. Gifford and C. T. Hull, 'Blood loss during and immediately after delivery', *Obstetrics and Gynaecology*, 17, 1961, pp. 9–18.

54. J. J. Nel, in *Episiotomy: Physical and Emotional Aspects*, National Childbirth Trust, 1972, p. 12.

55. S. Baker, *A Survey into Postnatal Perineal Discomfort*, Royal College of Midwives, London, 1971.

56. P. C. Buchan and J. A. J. Nicholls, *Journal of the Royal College of General Practitioners*, 30, 1980, pp. 297–300.

57. S. Kitzinger, in *Episiotomy: Physical and Emotional Aspects*, National Childbirth Trust, 1972, p. 19.

58. K. K. Shy and D. A. Essenbach, 'Fatal perineal cellulitis from an episiotomy site', *Obstetrics and Gynaecology*, 54(3), 1979.

59. E. Alberman, 'Facts and figures', in Chard and Richards, op. cit.

60. Suzanne Arms, op. cit.

61. F. M. Ettner, *Safe Alternatives in Childbirth*, NAPSAC Publications, 1975.

62. Suzanne Arms, op. cit., p. 83.

63. A. Blankfield, 'The optimum position for childbirth', *Medical Journal of Australia*, 16 October 1965, pp. 666–8.

64. J. Balaskas and A. Balaskas, *New Life*, Sidgwick & Jackson, 1979, ch. 4.

65. A. H. Kegel, 'Early genital relaxation', *Obstetrics and Gynaecology*, 8(5), 1956.

7 The third stage

1. W. M. O. Moore, in T. Chard and M. Richards (eds.), *Benefits and Hazards of the New Obstetrics*, Heinemann, 1977, p. 120.

2. M. C. Botha, 'The management of the umbilical cord in labour', *South African Journal of Obstetrics and Gynaecology*, 16(2), 1968, pp. 30–33.

3. M. M. Garrey *et al.*, *Obstetrics Illustrated*, Churchill Livingstone, Edinburgh, 1974, p. 498.

4. J. D. Paull and G. J. Ratten, *Medical Journal of Australia*, 1, 1977, p. 178.

5. Editorial, *Obstetric and Gynaecological Survey*, 12, 1957, p. 169.

6. W. J. Fitzgerald, *New York Medicine*, 58, 1958, p. 4081.

7. E. A. Cameron and E. B. French, *British Medical Journal*, 2, 1960, p. 28.

8. J. Chaasar Moir, *British Medical Journal*, 24 October 1964, pp. 1025–30.

9. A. C. Turnbull, *Postgraduate Medical Journal*, 5(Supplement), 1976, pp. 15–16.

10. B. Sorbe, *Obstetrics and Gynaecology*, 52(6), 1978.

11. D. J. Browning, 'Serious side effects of ergometrine and its use in routine obstetric practice', *Medical Journal of Australia*, 1, 1974, pp. 957–8.

12. E. A. Friedman, *American Journal of Obstetrics and Gynaecology*, 73, 1957, p. 1306.

13. J. D. Forman and R. L. Sullivan, *American Journal of Obstetrics and Gynaecology*, 63, 1952, p. 640.

14. C. A. D. Ringrose, *Canadian Medical Association Journal*, 87, 29 September 1962.

15. W. F. Howard *et al.*, *Journal of the American Medical Association*, 189(6), 10 August 1964.

16. N. F. Hacker and J. S. G. Briggs, *British Journal of Obstetrics and Gynaecology*, 86, August 1979, p. 633.

17. C. H. Hendricks and W. E. Brenner, *American Journal of Obstetrics and Gynaecology*, 108, 1970, p. 751.

18. D. W. J. Cullingford, correspondence, *British Medical Journal*, 10 August 1963, p. 386.

19. *Confidential Inquiry into Maternal Deaths*, HMSO, 1961–63.

20. P. Vardi, *Lancet*, 2, 1965, 12.

21. T. L. Montgomery, *Clinical Obstetrics and Gynaecology*, 3, 1960, pp. 900–910.

22. J. M. Gate, Correspondence, *British Medical Journal*, 1, 7 January 1978, p. 49.

23. L. Weinstein *et al.*, *Obstetrics and Gynaecology*, 37(1), 1971.

24. S. Z. Walsh, *Lancet*, 11 May 1968, pp. 996–7.

25. L. Snaith, *Journal of Obstetrics and Gynaecology of the British Empire*, 58, 1951, p. 633.

26. J. D. Martin and J. G. Dumoulin, *British Medical Journal*, 1, 1953, p. 643.

27. C. K. Vartan, *British Medical Journal*, 1, 1953, p. 1108.

28. C. J. Dewhurst and W. A. W. Dutton, *Lancet*, 19 October 1957, pp. 764–7.

29. J. R. Fliegner, *Medical Journal of Australia*, 26 August 1978, pp. 190–93.

30. M. Newton, L. Mosey, G. Egli, W. B. Gifford and C. T. Hull, *Obstetrics and Gynaecology*, 17, 1961, pp. 9–18.

31. E. A. Friedman, *American Journal of Obstetrics and Gynaecology*, 52, 1946, p. 746.
32. G. L. Clarke and C. P. Douglas, *Journal of Obstetrics and Gynaecology of the British Commonwealth*, 69, 1962, p. 404.
33. U. Neiminen and P. A. Järvinen, *Ann. Chir. Gynae.*, *Fenn.*, 53(4), 1964, pp. 424–9.
34. E. M. Greenberg, *American Journal of Obstetrics and Gynaecology*, 52, 1946, p. 746.
35. Association of Radical Midwives, Minutes of the meeting held in Boston, 26–28 October 1979.
36. S. Z. Walsh, *Lancet*, 11 May 1966, pp. 996–7.
37. J. H. Patterson, correspondence, *British Medical Journal*, 15 October 1966.
38. J. Munro Kerr and J. C. Moir, *Operative Obstetrics*, 5th edn. Ballière, Tindall & Cox, 1949, p. 807.
39. Margaret Mead and N. Newton, 'Cultural patterning of perinatal behaviour', in S. A. Richardson and A. F. Guttmacher (eds.), *Childbearing: Its Social and Psychological Aspects*, Williams & Wilkins, Baltimore, 1967.
40. C. S. Ford, 'A comparative study of human reproduction', *Yale University Publications in Anthropology*, no. 32, Yale University Press, New Haven, 1945.
41. Margaret Mead and N. Newton, op. cit., p. 144.
42. A. E. B. De Courcy-Wheeler, *British Medical Journal*, 18 August 1973.
43. M. C. Botha, *South African Journal of Obstetrics and Gynaecology*, 6(2), 24 August 1968, pp. 30–33.
44. C. Darwin, quoted by Louis Courtney, *British Medical Journal*, 28 July 1973, p. 236.
45. A. F. Meadows, *Manual of Midwifery*, 4th edn, Henry Renshaw, London, 1882, p. 192.
46. J. R. C. Burton-Brown, *Journal of Obstetrics and Gynaecology of the British Empire*, 56, 1949, pp. 847–55.
47. M. L. Brandt, *American Journal of Obstetrics and Gynaecology*, 23, 1933, pp. 662–7.
48. Györy and Damahidy, *Mschr. Geburtsh. Gynäk.*, 118, 1944, p. 192.
49. S. Z. Walsh, *Lancet*, 1, 1968, p. 996.
50. O. A. Lapido, *British Medical Journal*, 1, 1972, pp. 721–3.
51. P. M. Dunn, I. D. Frazer and A. B. Raper, *Journal of Obstetrics*

and Gynaecology of the British Commonwealth, 73, 1966, pp. 757–60.

52. J. E. Doolittle and C. R. Moritz, *Obstetrics and Gynaecology*, 27, 1966, p. 529; *Obstetrics and Gynaecology*, 22, 1963, p. 468.

53. L. Weinstein *et al.*, *Obstetrics and Gynaecology*, 37(1), 1971, pp. 70–73.

54. D. A. Berriman, *Midwives Chronicle and Nursing Notes*, March 1970.

55. G. L. Clarke and C. P. Douglas, *Journal of Obstetrics and Gynaecology of the British Commonwealth*, 69, 1962, p. 404.

56. T. L. Montgomery, *Clinical Obstetrics and Gynaecology*, 3, 1960, pp. 900–910.

57. A. J. Moss and M. Monset-Couchard, *Paediatrics*, 40(1), July 1967.

58. A. C. Yao and J. Lind, 'Placental transfusion', *American Journal of the Diseases of Childhood*, 127, 1974, pp. 128–41.

59. J. Lind, W. Oh and M. A. Oh, *Acta Paediatrica Scandanavica*, 56, 1966, p. 197.

60. P. Vardi, *Lancet*, 2, 1965, p. 12.

61. J. W. Williams, *Obstetrics*, 4th edn, D. Appleton, London, 1909, p. 298.

62. J. M. Gate, correspondence, *British Medical Journal*, 1, 7 January 1978, p. 49.

63. A. C. Yao and J. Lind, *Birth and the Family Journal*, 4(3), 1977, p. 91.

64. A. Redmond, S. Isana and D. Ingall, *Lancet*, 1, 1965, p. 283.

65. L. D. Courtney, *British Medical Journal*, 28 July 1973, p. 236.

66. A. J. Moss, E. D. Duffie and L. M. Fagan, *Journal of the American Medical Association*, 184, 1963, p. 48.

67. R. D. Laing, quoted in D. Brook, *Nature Birth*, Penguin, 1976, pp. 92–5.

68. M. Botha, *South African Journal of Obstetrics and Gynaecology*, 6(2), pp. 30–33.

69. M. L. Brandt, *American Journal of Obstetrics and Gynaecology*, 23, 1933, pp. 662–7.

70. J. H. Patterson, correspondence, *British Medical Journal*, 1, 1964, p. 377.

71. J. Barnes, 'Emergencies in general practice – postpartum maternal collapse', *British Medical Journal*, 28 May 1955, p. 1333.

72. B. M. Hibbard, *British Medical Journal*, 1, 1964, p. 1485.

73. M. E. Davis, 'Third-stage management', *American Journal of Surgery*, 48, 1940, p. 154.

74. J. R. Fliegner, *Medical Journal of Australia*, 26 August 1978, p. 193.

75. J. H. Patterson, correspondence, *British Medical Journal*, 31 August 1963, p. 563.

76. J. R. Fliegner and B. M. Hibbard, *British Medical Journal*, 10 September 1966, p. 623.

77. J. Kemp, correspondence, *British Medical Journal*, 31 August 1963, p. 563.

78. M. R. Fell, correspondence, *British Medical Journal*, 15 October 1966.

79. W. M. D. Moore, in Chard and Richards, op. cit., p. 120.

80. A. N. Cowan, correspondence, *British Medical Journal*, 10 August 1963, p. 387.

81. F. Leboyer, *Birth Without Violence*, A. Knopf, New York, 1975.

82. J. M. Weekley, *Obstetrics and Gynaecology News*, 1, 1 August 1975.

83. Anon., *Medical World News*, 16(10), 1975, pp. 22–30.

84. N. Whitley, *Journal of Nurse Midwifery*, 21, 1976, pp. 27–8.

85. A. MacFarlane, *The Psychology of Childbirth*, Fontana/Open Books, 1977, p. 19.

86. D. Walker *et al.*, 'Interuterine noise – a component of the foetal environment', *American Journal of Obstetrics and Gynaecology*, 109, 1971, pp. 91–5.

87. J. Lind, 'The family in the birth room', *Birth and the Family Journal*, 5(4), 1978, p. 25.

88. N. M. Nelson *et al.*, 'A randomized clinical trial of the Leboyer approach to childbirth', *New England Journal of Medicine*, 302, 1980, pp. 655–60.

89. L. S. Dahm and L. S. James, 'Newborn temperature and calculated heat loss in the delivery room', *Paediatrics*, 49(4), 1972, pp. 504–13.

90. D. Rappoport, *Bulletin psychologique*, 29, 1976, pp. 552–60.

91. G. Chamberlain *et al.*, *British Births 1970*, vol. 2: *Obstetric Care*, Heinemann, 1978.

92. D. Garrow, personal communication quoted in S. Kitzinger, *Birth at Home*, Oxford University Press, 1979, p. 40.

93. L. Cordero and E. Hon, 'Neonatal bradycardia following

nasopharyngeal stimulation', *Journal of Paediatrics*, 78(3), 1971, pp. 441–7.

94. M. Myles, *Textbook for Midwives*, Churchill Livingstone, Edinburgh, 1972, p. 310.

95. F. Leboyer, op. cit., p. 12.

96. R. Salter, *Medical News*, 12(44), 1980, p. 10.

97. C. Phillips, 'Neonatal heat loss in heat cribs v. mothers' arms', *Journal of the Nurses Association of the American College of Obstetricians and Gynaecologists*, 3(6), 1974.

98. M. Cornblath and R. Schwartz, *Disorders of Carbohydrate Metabolism in Infancy*, W. B. Saunders, Philadelphia, 1966.

99. J. M. Stephenson *et al.*, 'The effect of cooling on blood gas tensions in newly born human infants', quoted in Dahm and James, op. cit.

100. D. A. Fisher, T. H. Oddie, E. J. Makoski, *Paediatrics*, 37, 1966, p. 583.

101. L. Stern *et al.*, *Paediatrics*, 36, 1965, p. 367.

102. D. Schiff, L. Stern and J. Leduc, *Paediatrics*, 37, 1966, p. 577.

103. M. Klaus and J. Kennell, 'Human maternal behaviour at first contact with her young', *Paediatrics*, 46(2), 187–92.

104. A. MacFarlane, op. cit., p. 51.

105. D. Hales *et al.*, 'How early is early contact? Defining the limits of the sensitive period', *Paediatric Research*, 10, 1977, p. 448.

106. P. de Chateau *et al.*, *Birth and the Family Journal*, 3, Winter 1979, p. 149.

107. L. S. Dahm and L. S. James, op. cit.

108. A. MacLennan, Adelaide Hospital, personal communication, 1970.

109. S. Kitzinger, in Kitzinger and Davis, op. cit., p. 136.

110. S. O'Connor, K. B. Sherrod, H. M. Sandler and P. M. Vietze, *Birth and the Family Journal*, 5(4), 1978.

111. 'Parent–infant attachment', symposium reported in *Birth and the Family Journal*, 5(4), 1978.

112. S. Kitzinger, *Women as Mothers*, Fontana, 1978.

113. M. Klaus, 'The biology of parent-to-infant attachment', *Birth and the Family Journal*, 5(4), 1978, pp. 200–203.

114. A. MacFarlane, op. cit., p. 102.

115. H. Leiderman and M. Seashore, in A. MacFarlane, op. cit., p. 99.

116. M. Klaus and J. Kennell, 'Maternal attachment – importance

of the first postpartum days', *New England Journal of Medicine*, 286, 1972, p. 460.

117. D. Harvey, in *Breastfeeding Promotion Group News*, National Childbirth Trust, no. 11, November 1980, p. 10.
118. P. and A. Stanway, *Breast is Best*, Pan, 1978, p. 25.
119. C. Fisher, 'Successful breast feeding', in *Chatelaine's 'New Mother'* (ed. M. Istona), MacLean & Hunter, Toronto, 1980.

8 Alternatives and improvements

1. G. L. Kloosterman, 'The Dutch system of home births', in S. Kitzinger and J. Davis (eds.), *Place of Birth*, Oxford University Press, 1978, p. 90.
2. Suzanne Arms, *Immaculate Deception*, Houghton Mifflin, Boston, 1975, p. 277.
3. Suzanne Arms, op. cit., p. 264.
4. K. Newson, Minutes of the national meeting of the Association of Radical Midwives, 1–2 November 1980.
5. House of Commons Social Services Committee, Second Report, Session 1979/80, *Perinatal and Neonatal Mortality*, House of Commons Paper 663–1, HMSO, 1980.
6. S. Robinson, 'The vanishing midwife', *Nursing Times*, 24 April 1980, pp. 726–30.
7. G. L. Kloosterman, in Suzanne Arms, op. cit., p. 285.
8. M. Auld, *How Many Nurses?*, Royal College of Nursing Research Series, London, 1976.
9. J. Walker, 'Midwife or obstetric nurse? Some perceptions of midwives and obstetricians of the role of the midwife', *Journal of Advanced Nursing*, 1, 1976, pp. 129–38.
10. S. Robinson, Royal College of Midwives professional meeting paper, *Midwives Chronicle and Nursing Notes*, January 1981, pp. 11–15.
11. House of Commons Social Services Committee, op. cit., p. 72.
12. Suzanne Arms, op. cit., p. 255.
13. J. Willmott, 'Specialists in birth', *Nursing Mirror*, 17 July 1980, pp. 34–6.
14. *The Baby Killer: A War on Want Investigation into the Promotion and Sale of Powdered Baby Milks in the Third World*, War on Want, 467 Caledonian Road, London N7 9EB, 1974, p. 6.
15. R. C. Goodlin, 'Low-risk obstetric care for low-risk mothers', *Lancet*, 10 May 1980, p. 1017.

16. G. W. Taylor *et al.*, 'How safe is general practitioner obstetrics?', *Lancet*, 13 December 1980, p. 1287.
17. L. Mehl *et al.*, 'Home versus hospital delivery: comparison of matched populations', paper presented at the annual meeting of the American Public Health Association, Miami Beach, Florida, 20 October 1976.
18. S. Kitzinger, 'Women's experience of birth at home', in Kitzinger and Davis, op. cit., p. 135.
19. W. O. Goldthorpe and J. Richman, 'Reorganization of the maternity services: a comment on domiciliary confinment in view of the experience of the hospital strike, 1973', *Midwife and Health Visitor*, 10, 1974, pp. 265–70.
20. Association for the Improvement of Maternity Services, Editorial, *Newsletter*, June 1976.
21. Marjorie Tew, 'Facts, not assertions of belief', *Health and Social Services Journal*, 12 September 1980, pp. 1194–7.
22. P. Slack, 'Bricks without mortar', *Nursing Times*, 31 July 1980, pp. 1336–7.
23. M. Whitt, quoted in Suzanne Arms, op. cit. p. 213.
24. I. Chalmers, A. Oakley and A. MacFarlane, 'An immodest proposal', *British Medical Journal*, 22 March 1980, p. 842.
25. C. Fisher, personal communication, 1981.
26. C. Flint, 'A continuing labour of love', *Nursing Mirror*, 15 November 1979.

Appendix 2 Arranging a home birth

1. D. Ennals, *The Times*, 28 January 1978.
2. P. Jenkin, House of Commons Official Report, Parliamentary Debates (Hansard), 5 December 1980, vol. 995, no. 12, p. 810.
3. M. I. Stone, Presidential address, *American College of Obstetricians and Gynaecologists Newsletter*, 23(5), 1979, pp. 4–6.
4. N. Winterston, Short Report (Minutes of Evidence to the Social Services Committee), HMSO, 1980, p. 91.
5. V. Junor and M. Monaco, *Home Birth Handbook*, BIJA, The Old Convent, Beeches Green, Stroud, Glos., 1980, p. 54.
6. E. Alberman, 'Facts and figures', in T. Chard and M. Richards (eds.), *Benefits and Hazards of the New Obstetrics*, Heinemann, 1977.
7. G. Chamberlain *et al.*, *British Births 1970*, vol. 2: *Obstetric Care*, Heinemann, 1978.

8. G. L. Kloosterman, in Suzanne Arms, *Immaculate Deception*, Houghton Mifflin, Boston, 1975, p. 287.

Appendix 4 Coping with perineal stitches: Some practical advice

1. E. Montgomery, *Episiotomy: Physical and Emotional Aspects*, National Childbirth Trust, 1972, p. 2.
2. C. Fieldhouse, 'Treatment note: ultrasound for relief of painful episiotomy scars', *Physiotherapy*, 65(7), 1979.

Appendix 5 The cascade of intervention

1. M. Blancow, M. N. Smith, M. Graham and R. G. Wilson, *Lancet*, 1, 1975, p. 217.
2. I. Chalmers, H. Campbell and A. C. Turnbull, *British Medical Journal*, 2, 1975, p. 116.
3. A. A. Calder and M. P. Embury, 'The management of labour', *Proceedings of the Royal College of Obstetricians and Gynaecologists Third Study Group*, 64, 1975.
4. W. A. Liston and A. J. Campbell, *British Medical Journal*, 3, 1974, p. 606.
5. M. P. M. Richards, *Early Human Development*, 1, 1977, p. 3.
6. I. Chalmers, J. G. Lawson and A. C. Turnbull, *British Journal of Obstetrics and Gynaecology*, 83, 1976, p. 921.
7. J. Arroyo and C. J. Mendez-Bauer, *Perinatal Medicine*, 3, 1975, p. 129.
8. I. J. Hoult, A. H. MacLennan and L. E. S. Carrie, *British Medical Journal*, 1, 1977, p. 14.
9. P. R. S. Brinsden and A. D. Clark, *British Medical Journal*, 2, 1978, pp. 855–6.
10. P. Yudkin, A. M. Frumar, A. B. M. Anderson and A. C. Turnbull, *British Journal of Obstetrics and Gynaecology*, 'A retrospective study of induction of labour', 86(4), 1979, pp. 257–65.
11. M. Newton, L. Mosey, G. E. Egli, W. B. Gifford and C. T. Hull, 'Blood loss during and immediately after delivery', *Obstetrics and Gynaecology*, 17, 1961, pp. 9–18.
12. M. A. Lyon, *Lancet*, 2, 1975, p. 317.
13. E. A. Friedman, M. R. Sachtleben and B. A. Bresky, *American Journal of Obstetrics and Gynaecology*, 127, 1977, p. 779.

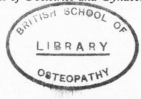

Index

ABO incompatability, *see* isoimmunization
acceleration of labour, 36, 79–81
admission procedures, 39, 43–7
adrenalin, 237
afterbirth, *see* placenta
age, risk factors, 28–9
Ahlfeld, 173
ambulation, 47–52
American Foundation for Maternal and Child Health, 66
amnion, 82
aminoscopy, 58, 77
amniotic fluid, function of, 82, 211
  rupture of membranes, 56–8, 212
amniotomy, acceleration of labour, 79, 81, 82, 86
  early *v.* late rupture, 83–6
  in induced labour, 56–8, 59, 61, 62, 63
  reasons for, 82–3
anaesthesia, general, 53–4, 174
  local, 107–16
  spinal, 116
  see also epidural anaesthesia
analgesics, *see* drugs
Anderson, 66
antenatal care, 32, 198
  in Holland, 192–3
  home births, 223
  midwives' involvement in, 200

antepartum haemorrhage, 30, 74, 115, 146
anti-D immunoglobulin, *see* rhesus disease
antibiotics, penicillin-resistant bacteria, 226
  use of after membrane rupture, 212
antibodies, *see* rhesus disease
Apgar scoring, 67–8
Arabs, 19
Arms, Suzanne, 124
Ashford, J. R., 27
Association of Radical Midwives, 16, 218
attachment, mother/baby, 181–90
Aucher, Marie Louise, 236–7
auscultation, 89–91
Austria, 23

back pain, 121
Banta, D., 91
Bantus, 145–6, 171
barbituates, 104
Barnes, Dame Josephine, 173
bathing babies after delivery, 177
bearing down, 113, 123–9
Beasley, 66
Bedford, G. S., 44
belladonna, 20
Berriman, D. A., 165
Berry, R. J., 33

Beynon, Constance, 126, 127
Biggs, J. S. G., 150, 154
bilirubin, 69, 168, 189
Birmingham Maternity Hospital, 54
birth chairs and stools, 22, 48, 122
bladder, complications following
    epidural anaesthesia, 114
Blankfield, Adele, 119–20, 124–5, 142
bleeding, 57
    see also antepartum haemorrhage;
        postpartum haemhorrhage
blood pressure, birth positions and,
    49–50
    effect of epidural anaesthesia on,
        112–13
    effect of ergometrine on, 150–1, 154
    lowered, 112–13
    raised, 30, 70, 111
    in second stage, 125
    see also supine hypotension
blood sampling, foetal, 87
Boissonnas, 148
bonding, 185–6
    see also attachment
Bonham, D. G., 76
Botha, M. C., 145–6, 163–4, 171, 175
Boucher, 21
Bourgeois, Louise, 20–1
bowels, enemas and suppositories, 39,
    46–7, 224, 229, 233
Brackbill, Y, 104
brain damage, 84–5, 153
Brandsel, C., 136–7
Brandt, 174
Braun, 133
Braxton Hicks contractions, 210, 213
Brazelton, 185
breaking the waters, see membranes
breast-feeding, 189–90, 205–6, 225
breath-holding, in second stage, 123–5
breathing problems, 66–9, 72, 105, 179
breech delivery, 30, 133, 134, 239
Brindsen, P. R. S., 65
British Birth Survey, 222
British Medical Journal, 94, 168, 175
British Perinatal Mortality Survey, 29
British Postgraduate Medical
    Federations, 34
Browning, D. J., 150
Buchan, P. C., 139
Budin, 168
Bull, Dr, 216–17
Burchell, R., 45

Burns, J., 133
Butler, N. R., 76, 85, 128
The Byrth of Mankynde, 20

Caesarian section, 39, 70, 240
    in diabetic pregnancies, 73
    and electronic foetal monitoring, 89,
        90–1
    foetal distress, 66
    following pre-eclampsia, 71
    in induced labour, 64–5
    in prolonged labour, 79, 81
    subsequent pregnancies, 29, 61
    using epidural anaesthesia, 111
Caldeyro-Barcia, Dr R., 66, 83–4, 127,
    141
Campbell, A. J., 66
caput succedaneum, 51, 84
Carmichael, J. H. E., 33
Central Midwives Board, 23, 133, 196,
    215
cervix, dilatation, 95
    and rupture of membranes, 57, 58
    stimulation of, 56, 58
Chalmers, I., 135, 207
Chamberlen, Hugh, 22
Chamberlen, Peter, 21
Chateau, Peter de, 185
chorion, 82
Church, attitude to medicine, 18–20
Church of England, 21
Churchill, F., 44
Clarke, A. D., 65
Clarke, G. L., 155, 159
Clément, Jules, 21
Cohen, W. R., 128
Colbert, Jean, 21
community midwives, 200, 201, 203–6,
    218, 221
contact, see attachment
contractions, and baby's heart rate,
    86–7
    bearing down, 127–8
    during pregnancy, 210, 213
    early stages, 212–13
    expectation of pain, 95–100
    first stage, 213
    in induced labour, 63–4
    and rupture of membranes, 86
    second stage, 213, 214
cord, see umbilical cord
Courtney, Dr L. D., 169
Crede, 172–3

crowning, 214

Dahm, L. S., 182–3
Darwin, Erasmus, 161
Davies, 168
de Courcy-Wheeler, Dr, 160
De Lee, J. B., 43, 127
delivery rooms, 55
  temperature of, 177, 181, 182, 227
Demerol, *see* pethidine
Denman, T., 44
Denmark, midwifery in, 194–5, 198, 208
  perinatal mortality, 16
de Vault, S., 35
Dewees, William Pott, 48, 117, 161
Dewhurst, 152–3
diabetes, 30, 70, 72–3, 111
diaphragm, 125
diarrhoea, 47
diazepam, 106
dilatation, *see* cervix
doctors, relations with midwives, 198, 200–1
Donnison, Jean, 16
Doolittle, J. E., 164–5
Douglas, C. P., 155, 159
Douglas, Dr John, 22
drugs, in accelerated labour, 81
  and expectation of pain, 93–4
  as a first line of defence, 98
  historical use of, 20
  and hypoxia, 68
  management of third stage, 145–59
  and mother/baby interaction, 187–8
  side-effects, 101–2
  as a substitute for emotional support, 98–9
  use of in labour, 100–16
Duffie, E. D., 169
Dunn, Peter, 35–6, 98
Du Vigneaud, 148

eating and drinking, in labour, 52–4
eclampsia, 151
Edinburgh, 22
Egypt, ancient, 22
Elder, M. G., 62
endorphins, 237
enemas, 39, 46–7, 224, 229, 233
Engelmann, G. J., 48–9
Enkin, Dr Murrary, 39–40
Ennals, Dr David, 215

Entonox, 106–7
epidural anaesthesia, advantages and disadvantages, 111–16
  effects on baby, 104
  episiotomy, 144
  in induced labour, 64, 65
  methods of administration, 108–10
  reasons for, 100
  supine hypotension, 49–50
episiotomy, 118, 130–44
  healing, 137, 241–3
  home births, 224–5
  perineal shaving, 43, 45
  prevention of, 128, 141–4, 239
  reasons for, 133–7
  side-effects, 137–40
  stitches, 128, 138–40, 234, 241–3
ergometrine, 145–7, 148–59, 165, 171, 221
ergot of rye, 20, 147
ergotamine, 147
ergotoxine, 147
essential hypertension, 70

Fagan, L. M., 169
false labour, 213
fathers, *see* husbands
fear, effect on labour, 38–9
  expectation of pain in labour, 96–7
Fentazin, 106
fibroids, 29
Finland, perinatal mortality, 205
first baby, *see* primagravida
first stage, 55, 56–116
Flexner Report, 24
Fliegner, J. R., 174
Flint, Caroline, 208
fluid retention, 30
'flying squads', 156, 222
foetal bradycardia, 115
foetal distress, 70
  in induced labour, 63, 65, 66
  prediction of, 77–8
foetal growth retardation, 30–1, 70–1, 73–4, 75
foetal monitoring, 34–5, 36, 58
  advantages and disadvantages, 88–92
  and amniotomy, 82–3
  during induction, 63
  methods of, 86–8
foetal-movement counts, 76, 77–8
food and drink, during labour, 52–4
forceps delivery, 39, 128–9

association with jaundice, 69
episiotomy, 133, 134
foetal distress, 66
in induced labour, 64–5
mother's position, 48, 119–20
and use of epidural anaesthesia,
    113–14, 116
forewaters, 56–7, 211
Forman, J. D., 150
fourth (or subsequent) baby, *see*
    multigravida
France, development of midwifery,
    20–2, 23
Odent method of delivery, 236–40
Franklin, Dr A. W., 41
Fredric, J., 85
Friedman, E. A., 150, 154–5
Fryer, J. G., 27
fundal pressure, 129–30, 149, 164, 173

Galen, 19
Garrow, Dr Donald, 179
'gas and air', 106–7
general practitioner units, 203
Germany, 20, 24
glomerular nephritis, *see* renal disease
glucose, 52–3, 54
glycogen, 52–3
Goldthorpe, W. O., 206
Goodlin, R. C., 206
Gordon, M., 86
Gordon-Wright, A. P., 62
growth retardation, 30–1, 70–1, 73–4,
    75

habituation, 104, 105
Hacker, N. F., 150, 154
haemorrhage, antepartum, 30, 74, 115,
    146
    postpartum, 30, 65–6, 145–7,
    149–50, 154–9, 161, 163–4, 175,
    221
Hall, M., 75
Harvey, William, 21
Haverkamp, A. D., 89–90
head (baby's), caput succedaneum, 51,
    84
    moulding, 51, 84–5
Head, Sir Henry, 94
heart rate (foetal), effect of epidural
    anaesthesia on, 115
    monitoring, 86–92
    and rupture of membranes, 85–6

in second stage, 127
height, risk factors, 29
herbal remedies, 20
Hibbard, B. M., 174
hindwaters, 56–7, 211–12
hip joints, 180
Hippocrates, 18
Holland, episiotomy rate, 141
    home births, 28, 194, 222
    midwifery in, 23, 192–4
    perinatal mortality, 16, 205
    use of drugs in labour, 93
Homburg, R., 77
home births, advantages, 219–20,
    223–6
    conduct of, 233–5
    disadvantages, 221–2
    effects on mothers, 37–8
    intervention in, 36–7
    and perinatal mortality, 27–8, 31–3
    preparation for, 215–18, 227–33
home helps, 215
hospital deliveries, admission
    procedures, 39, 43–7
    advantages, 219, 220
    delivery rooms, 55
    disadvantages, 220–1
    effects on mothers, 37–42
    and mother/baby interaction, 188–90
    obstetric interference, 33–6
    and perinatal mortality, 26–33
Hottentots, 52
House, 137
Howard, F., 118, 119, 120, 150, 153–4
husbands, home births, 225
    supportive role, 39–40
hyaluronidase, 149
hypertension, 30, 70, 111
hyperventilation, 100, 107
hypoglycaemia, 181
hypothermia, 106
hypotonia, 106
hypoxia, 68, 79, 115, 126–7
hysterotomy, 29

iatrogenic contamination, 44
idiopathic respiratory distress, 169
induction, 36
    benefits, 69–73
    diabetic pregnancies, 73
    disadvantages to baby, 66–9
    disadvantages to mother, 62–6
    enemas and, 46–7

methods, 56–62
placental insufficiency, 73–9
home v. hospital births, 225–6
intrauterine, 57
inhalation analgesia, 106–7
intravenous feeding, 53
intubation, 67
iron tablets, 193
Islam, 19
isoimmunization, 29, 70, 71–2, 164–5
Italy, 19

James I, King of England, 21
James, L. S., 182–3
jaundice, 69, 152, 168, 189
Jeffcoate, T. N. A., 127
Jenkin, Patrick, 215–16
Johnston, R. A., 44, 45
Junor, V., 218

Kantor, H., 45
Kelso, I. M., 89–91
Kennell, J., 181–2, 186
Kerr, M. G., 49
ketones, 53
ketosis, 53, 54
kidney disease, 30, 70–1
Kitzinger, Sheila, 183–4, 206
Klaus, Marshall, 181–2, 184–5, 186
Kloosterman, G. L., 16, 35, 197
Krämer, Heinrich, 20
Kurjak, 66

labour, acceleration, 36, 79–81
amniotomy, 82–6
bearing down, 123–9
beginnings of, 210–13
delivery rooms, 55
eating and drinking during, 52–4
expectation of pain, 93–100
first stage, 55, 56–116
length of, 50, 51
methods of pain relief, 100–16
mother's position during, 47–52
preterm, 70
prolonged, 79–81, 97–8
second stage, 55, 117–44
third stage, 145–75
transition stage, 55, 213
see also induction
Lapido, O. A., 165
Laing, R. D., 170
Lancet, 98

Lankford, H., 44
la Vallière, Louise de, 21
Leak, 142
Leboyer, Dr Frederick, 175–8, 180, 236
Leeson, J., 74
Leiderman, H., 186
levallorphan, 105
Lewis, Sir Thomas, 97
Lind, J., 167–9, 177
liquor amni, see amniotic fluid
Lister, Joseph, 24
Liston, W. A., 66
lithotomy position, 48, 117–23, 141–2
local anaesthetic, episiotomy, 137–8
Lomas, P., 45
Loncier, Adam, 147
Louis XIV, King of France, 21
low back pain, 121
low birth weight babies, 30
Lusk, W. T., 49, 118

McDonald, J. S., 115
Macfarlane, A., 182, 185–6, 207
MacLennan, A., 78
McMaster University Medical Center, 177, 178
McNay, M.B., 74
Malleus Maleficarum, 19–20
Manus, 52, 160
Marie de' Medici, 21
Martin, 69
massage, uterine, 155
maternal deaths, 26–7
in epidural anaesthesia, 113
and ergometrine, 151, 156
following episiotomy, 140
postpartum haemorrhage, 146, 161
in prolonged labour, 79
maternal illnesses, 70–3
maternity aid nurses, 193
Mather, 34
Mauriceau, François, 21–2, 48, 171
Mead, Margaret, 16, 35, 160
Meadows, A. F., 161
meconium, 57, 77
Mehl, L., 136–7, 206
membranes, artificial rupture of, see amniotomy
function of, 82
spontaneous rupture of, 83, 212
men-midwives, 21–2
Mendez–Bauer, C. J., 50, 119

Mengert, 122–3
meperidine, *see* pethidine
Merriman, S., 48, 52, 133
Michaelis, 132–3
midwifery, in Britain, 21, 22–3, 24–5, 195–209
    decline of, 15–16
    in Denmark, 194–5, 198, 208
    development of, 18–25
    in Holland, 23, 192–4
    home births, 208, 217–18, 223–5, 227–35
    licencing, 23, 24
Midwives Acts, 16, 23, 24–5, 196, 208, 215
Midwives Institute, 23
Moir, Dr J. Chassar, 147, 148, 159
Monaco, M., 218
monitoring, *see* foetal monitoring
Montespan, Madame de, 21
Montgomery, T. L., 151, 166, 167
Moritz, C. R., 164–5
Morley, Dr David, 206
morphine, 102
mortality, *see* maternal deaths; perinatal mortality
Moss, A. J., 167, 169
moulding, of baby's head, 51, 84–5
Mowbray, Dr John, 22
mucus extraction, 179–80
mucus plug, 210–11
Muller, P. F., 85
multigravida, risk factors, 29
Murphy, 122–3
Myles, M., 43
myomectomy, 29

Naaktgeboren, C., 97
Naroll, F., 118, 122
National Center for Health Care (USA), 91
National Childbirth Trust, 204
National Institute of Health (USA), 88, 91
National Perinatal Epidemiology Unit, 32
Navaho Indians, 93
navel, 166
neonatal ophthalmia, 24
nesting activity, 210
New Haven Medical Center, 179–80
Newton, F., 119, 120, 122, 154, 155
Nicholls, J. A. J., 139

Nigeria, 206
nipple soreness, 189–90
Niswander, K. R., 86
nitrazine sticks, 212
Northwick Park Hospital, Middlesex, 43–4
Norway, 16, 23
Nurses, Midwives and Health Visitors Act (1979), 25
Nursing Education Research Unit, 199

Oakley, Dr Ann, 32, 207
Obstetrical Society of London, 23
Odent, Dr Michel, 236–40
O'Driscoll, K., 34, 71, 73, 75, 81
oedema, 30
oestriol levels, 75, 77–8
Oh, M. A., 167–8
Oh, W., 167–8
operations, uterine, 29
Ould, Sir Fielding, 132
overbreathing, 100, 107
overdue pregnancies, 76–7
oxytocin, acceleration of labour, 79–81
    association with jaundice, 69
    challenge tests, 77
    discovery of, 148
    and foetal distress, 66
    in induced labour, 56, 57, 58–60, 62
    natural release of, 237
    and respiratory depression, 66–8
    side-effects, 62, 64, 65–6
    in third stage of labour, 148, 153–9, 163, 165, 168

pain, expectation of, 93–100
    in induced labour, 64
    medieval attitudes to, 20
    and mother's position, 50, 51, 118–19
    relief by drugs, 100–16
    and rupture of membranes, 86
paracervical block, 108
Paré, Ambroise, 20–1
Paris, Hôtel-Dieu, 20–1
Pasteur, Louis, 24
Patterson, J. H., 158, 172, 173, 175
Paull, J. D., 146, 159
Peel report, 26, 198–9, 200, 206
pelvic-floor exercises, 143–4, 241
pelvis, size, 29
Pennoyer, 129
Penthrane, 106–7

perinatal mortality, 16
  and diabetes, 72–3
  electronic foetal monitoring and, 87
  home v. hospital births, 216–17, 221, 222
  and induction, 74–5
  and pre-eclampsia, 76
  respiratory distress, 69
  risk factors, 26–33
  and use of midwives, 205
perineum, episiotomy, 130–44
  shaving, 39, 43–5, 223–4
  stitches, 128, 138–40, 234, 241–3
  tears, 118, 119, 121, 130, 134–5, 137, 144
perphenazine, 106
Peterson, G., 136–7
pethidine, 64, 67, 101, 102–5
pethilorphan, 104, 105
Phenergan, 106
phenothiazine, 106
phototherapy, 69, 189
Pithiviers, Centre Hospitalier General, 236–40
pituitary gland, 58, 59, 148
placenta, delayed delivery of, 162–3
  delivery of, 120, 129, 145–6, 149, 239
  and hypertension, 70, 71
  malfunction, 31
  manual removal of, 152, 159, 163, 172, 174
  methods of delivery, 170–5
  placental insufficiency, 73–9
  retained, 30, 145–6, 147, 155, 156, 163
  separation of, 152, 156, 161–3, 170
polyhydramnios, 72, 73
position (of baby), malpresentation, 30
position (of mother), during induced labour, 62–3
  in labour, 22, 47–52, 238–9
  lithotomy position, 117–23
  and pain, 94
  and prevention of tears and episiotomies, 141–2
postnatal blues, 226
postpartum haemorrhage, 30, 65–6, 145–7, 149–50, 154–9, 161, 163–4, 175, 221
pre-eclampsia, 30, 70, 71, 72, 76, 106, 111
preterm delivery, 70

primagravida, risk factors, 28
prolactin, 148
prolapse, umbilical cord, 212
  uterus, 126, 141, 172, 174
prolonged labour, 79–81
prolonged pregnancy, 76–7
promazine, 106
promethazine, 106
prostaglandin, 56, 58, 60–2
proteinuria, 30, 70, 71
pubic hair, shaving, 39, 43–5
pudendal nerve block, 107–8, 111, 116
puerpural sepsis, 21, 24, 43
pushing, 113, 123–9

Queen Charlotte's Hospital, 189

Radcliffe Infirmary, Oxford, 32
Rappoport, D., 177
Ratten, G. J., 146, 159
Read, Grantly Dick, 96, 97–8
Reformation, 21
Reich, Wilhelm, 236
relaxation classes, 98
renal disease, 30, 70–1
Renou, 89–90
respiratory depression, 66–9, 105
respiratory distress syndrome, 68–9, 72
rhesus disease, 29, 70, 71–2, 164–5
Richards, Martin, 68, 103, 105
Richman, J., 206
Rigshospital, Copenhagen, 194
Ringrose, C. A. D., 150, 156
risk factors, 28–3, 216
Rosen, M., 108
Rosengreen, W. R., 35
Royal College of Midwives, 23, 24–5, 196, 218
Russell, J. G. B., 121
Russia, 23

safety, home births, 221–3
  hospital deliveries, 26–8, 206, 220
St Anthony's fire, 147
Salter, Dr Robert, 180
Schneider, J., 77
Schwarcz, R., 51
Schwartz, Phillip, 85
Scotland, 22
Scott, D. B., 49
Seashore, M., 186
Semmelweis, Ignaz Philipp, 24
separation, of mother and baby, 183–90
  of the mother from her family, 37–42

septicaemia, 172
shaving, perineal, 39, 43–5
Short Committee, 221
show, 210–11
Sidall, R. S., 44, 45
sitting, delivery posture, 122–3, 159
Slack, Pamela, 208–9
sleep, after delivery, 188
Smellie, William, 22, 49
Smith, A., 74
social class, and mother/child bonding, 186
   risk factors, 29
Social Services Committee, 202, 206–8
Society of Apothecaries, 22
Society for the Support of Home
   Confinements, 217, 218
Soranus of Ephesus, 18, 20
Sorbe, B., 155
Spain, 19
Sparine, 106
Spastic Society, 32
spinal anaesthesia, 116
Sprenger, Jakob, 20
squatting, delivery position, 121, 145, 239
staphylococcus aureous, 226
Stearns, John, 147
stitches, perineal, 128, 138–40, 234, 241–3
stress, effect on labour, 38–9
stress incontinence, 126
sucking ability, effects of drugs on, 104, 106
   effect of epidural anaesthesia on, 115
sugar, in urine, 52–3
Sullivan, R. L., 150
supine hypotension, 49–50, 113
suppositories, 39, 46–7, 224, 233
Sweden, midwives, 23
   perinatal mortality, 16, 205
Syntocinon, 59, 60, 148, 156, 158
syntometrine, 145–7, 149–53, 156, 158, 170–2, 221

Taylor, G. W., 206
temperature, of babies, 177, 181, 182–3
   of delivery room, 177, 181, 182, 227
Tew, Marjorie, 27–8, 32, 206
Thacker, S., 91
third stage, 145–75
This, Bernard, 236
thumb-sucking, 105

toxaemia, 30, 111
tranquillizers, 104, 106
transition period, 55, 213
Turnbull, A. C., 66
twins, 153

ultrasound, scanning, 33, 75–6
   treatment of episiotomy scars, 242–3
umbilical cord, 159–70
   clamping, 151–2, 160–1, 163–70
   compression, 85–6
   cutting, 157, 160, 165
   milking, 167
   prolapse, 212
   pulling on, 149, 157, 158–9, 171–5
United States of America, foetal
   monitoring, 34–5
   midwives, 15, 16, 23–4
   perinatal mortality, 205
urine, protein in, 30, 70, 71
   sugar in, 52–3
uterus, effect of enemas on, 46–7
   inefficiency, 79
   inversion, 126, 141, 172, 174
   muscles, 95–6
   nerves, 95–6
   operations on, 29
   retraction, 161–2

vacuum extraction, 116, 128–9, 240
vagina, damage to, 125–6
   examinations, 39
vaginal tablets, induction, 62
Valium, 106
Valsalva manoeuvre, 125
Vardi, P., 168
Vaughan, K. O., 121

Walker, J., 200
Walsh, S. Z., 163, 164, 175
Warren, S. P., 44
water, babies born in, 238
waters, see amniotic fluid
weight, low birth weight, 30
   maternal weight gain, 31
Weinstein, L., 165
Wennberg, J., 87
Whitt, Michael, 207
Williams, J. W., 44–5, 168
witchcraft, 19–20
World Health Organization, 34

X-rays in pregnancy, 33

Yao, A. C., 167, 168–9